DSM-5-TR Diagnostic Handbook

1000+ Interactive Questions, Real-World Scenarios, and Practical Diagnostic Guides

James K. Alston

Contents

SECTION 1: INTRODUCTION TO DSM-5-TR AND CLINICAL DIAGNOSIS 8

CHAPTER 1: INTRODUCTION TO DSM-5-TR 8

   1.1 KEY UPDATES IN DSM-5-TR 8
   1.2 PURPOSE OF DSM-5-TR IN CLINICAL DIAGNOSIS 9

CHAPTER 2: HOW TO USE THIS BOOK 11

   2.1 USING INTERACTIVE QUESTIONS 11
   2.2 APPLYING REAL-WORLD CLINICAL CASES...12
   2.3 UTILIZING STEP-BY-STEP DIAGNOSTIC GUIDES..13
   2.4 PRACTICAL APPLICATION AND STUDY TIPS 15

CHAPTER 3: DIAGNOSTIC TOOLS AND ICD-10-CM CODES...17

   3.1 OVERVIEW OF DIAGNOSTIC TOOLS 17
   3.2 DSM-5-TR AND ICD-10-CM CRITERIA MAPPING 19
   3.3 PRACTICAL AND INSURANCE USE OF ICD-10-CM CODES 20

SECTION 2: 1000+ INTERACTIVE QUESTIONS TO TEST YOUR KNOWLEDGE 23

CHAPTER 4: NEURODEVELOPMENTAL DISORDERS...23

   4.1 ADHD 23
   4.2 AUTISM SPECTRUM DISORDER 24
   4.3 INTELLECTUAL DISABILITIES 26
   4.4 COMMUNICATION DISORDERS...27
   4.5 SPECIFIC LEARNING DISORDERS 29
   4.6 MOTOR DISORDERS 30

CHAPTER 5: SCHIZOPHRENIA SPECTRUM AND OTHER PSYCHOTIC DISORDERS 32

   5.1 SCHIZOPHRENIA...32
   5.2 SCHIZOAFFECTIVE DISORDER 33
   5.3 DELUSIONAL DISORDER..34
   5.4 BRIEF PSYCHOTIC DISORDER 36
   5.5 CATATONIA 37

CHAPTER 6: BIPOLAR AND RELATED DISORDERS 39

   6.1 BIPOLAR I DISORDER 39
   6.2 BIPOLAR II DISORDER 40
   6.3 CYCLOTHYMIC DISORDER..41
   6.4 SUBSTANCE/MEDICATION-INDUCED BIPOLAR DISORDER 43
   6.5 OTHER SPECIFIED BIPOLAR DISORDERS 44

CHAPTER 7: DEPRESSIVE DISORDERS 46

7.1 MAJOR DEPRESSIVE DISORDER 46

7.2 PERSISTENT DEPRESSIVE DISORDER (DYSTHYMIA) 47

7.3 DISRUPTIVE MOOD DYSREGULATION DISORDER..48

7.4 PREMENSTRUAL DYSPHORIC DISORDER 50

7.5 SUBSTANCE/MEDICATION-INDUCED DEPRESSIVE DISORDER 51

CHAPTER 8: ANXIETY DISORDERS 53

8.1 GENERALIZED ANXIETY DISORDER 53

8.2 PANIC DISORDER 54

8.3 SPECIFIC PHOBIAS 55

8.4 SOCIAL ANXIETY DISORDER 56

8.5 AGORAPHOBIA 58

8.6 SEPARATION ANXIETY DISORDER 59

CHAPTER 9: OBSESSIVE-COMPULSIVE AND RELATED DISORDERS 61

9.1 OBSESSIVE-COMPULSIVE DISORDER...61

9.2 BODY DYSMORPHIC DISORDER 62

9.3 HOARDING DISORDER 63

9.4 TRICHOTILLOMANIA (HAIR-PULLING DISORDER) 65

9.5 EXCORIATION (SKIN-PICKING) DISORDER 66

CHAPTER 10: TRAUMA- AND STRESSOR-RELATED DISORDERS.. 68

10.1 POST-TRAUMATIC STRESS DISORDER (PTSD)..68

10.2 ACUTE STRESS DISORDER 69

10.3 ADJUSTMENT DISORDERS 70

10.4 REACTIVE ATTACHMENT DISORDER 72

10.5 DISINHIBITED SOCIAL ENGAGEMENT DISORDER..73

CHAPTER 11: SOMATIC SYMPTOM AND RELATED DISORDERS.. 75

11.1 SOMATIC SYMPTOM DISORDER 75

11.2 ILLNESS ANXIETY DISORDER 76

11.3 CONVERSION DISORDER (FUNCTIONAL NEUROLOGICAL SYMPTOM DISORDER)................77

11.4 FACTITIOUS DISORDER 79

CHAPTER 12: OTHER CATEGORIES OF DISORDERS 81

12.1 SLEEP-WAKE DISORDERS...81

12.2 PERSONALITY DISORDERS 82

12.3 NEUROCOGNITIVE DISORDERS 83

12.4 FEEDING AND EATING DISORDERS 85

12.5 SEXUAL DYSFUNCTIONS...86

12.6 GENDER DYSPHORIA..87

12.7 DISRUPTIVE, IMPULSE-CONTROL, AND CONDUCT DISORDERS 88

12.8 SUBSTANCE-RELATED AND ADDICTIVE DISORDERS 89

ANSWERS TO INTERACTIVE QUESTIONS 91

SECTION 3: REAL-WORLD CLINICAL CASES 92

INTRODUCTION TO SECTION 3: THE VALUE OF CASE STUDIES IN CLINICAL PRACTICE 92

CHAPTER 13: CLINICAL CASES IN NEURODEVELOPMENTAL DISORDERS **94**

13.0 Introduction to Neurodevelopmental Disorders 94
Case 13.1: Autism Spectrum Disorder 95
Case 13.2: Attention-Deficit/Hyperactivity Disorder (ADHD) 97
Case 13.3: Intellectual Disability 100
Case 13.4: Communication Disorder 103
Case 13.5: Specific Learning Disorder 106

CHAPTER 14: CLINICAL CASES IN SCHIZOPHRENIA AND OTHER PSYCHOTIC DISORDERS **109**

14.0 Introduction to Psychotic Disorders 109
Case 14.1: Schizophrenia 110
Case 14.2: Schizoaffective Disorder 113
Case 14.3: Brief Psychotic Disorder 116
Case 14.4: Delusional Disorder 119
Case 14.5: Catatonia 122

CHAPTER 15: CLINICAL CASES IN BIPOLAR AND RELATED DISORDERS **125**

15.0 Introduction to Bipolar and Related Disorders 125
Case 15.1: Bipolar I Disorder 126
Case 15.2: Bipolar II Disorder 129
Case 15.3: Cyclothymic Disorder 132
Case 15.4: Substance/Medication-Induced Bipolar Disorder 135
Case 15.5: Bipolar Disorder with Comorbid Anxiety 138

CHAPTER 16: CLINICAL CASES IN DEPRESSIVE DISORDERS. **141**

16.0 Introduction to Depressive Disorders 141
Case 16.1: Major Depressive Disorder 142
Case 16.2: Persistent Depressive Disorder (Dysthymia) 145
Case 16.3: Depression with Psychotic Features 148
Case 16.4: Postpartum Depression 151
Case 16.5: Substance-Induced Depressive Disorder 154

CHAPTER 17: CLINICAL CASES IN ANXIETY DISORDERS **157**

17.0 Introduction to Anxiety Disorders 157
Case 17.1: Generalized Anxiety Disorder 158
Case 17.2: Panic Disorder 161
Case 17.3: Social Anxiety Disorder 164
Case 17.4: Agoraphobia 167
Case 17.5: Separation Anxiety Disorder 170

CHAPTER 18: CLINICAL CASES IN TRAUMA- AND STRESSOR-RELATED DISORDERS **173**

18.0 Introduction to Trauma- and Stressor-Related Disorders 173
Case 18.1: Post-Traumatic Stress Disorder (PTSD) 174
Case 18.2: Acute Stress Disorder 177
Case 18.3: Adjustment Disorder 179
Case 18.4: Reactive Attachment Disorder 182
Case 18.5: Trauma-Induced Dissociative Disorder 185

SECTION 4: PRACTICAL DIAGNOSTIC GUIDES AND QUICK REFERENCE TOOLS 188

INTRODUCTION TO SECTION 4 188

CHAPTER 19: DIAGNOSTIC GUIDES FOR COMPLEX CASES 189

19.1 DIAGNOSTIC AND MANAGEMENT APPROACHES FOR COMORBID DISORDERS 189
19.2 EVALUATING SYMPTOM SEVERITY 190
19.3 RISK ASSESSMENT IN COMPLEX CASES 193

CHAPTER 20: DIFFERENTIAL DIAGNOSIS AND DECISION-MAKING TOOLS 196

20.1 SYMPTOM OVERLAP: TABLES AND GUIDES 196
20.2 DECISION TREES AND DIAGNOSTIC ALGORITHMS 199
20.3 STRATEGIES FOR DIFFERENTIAL DIAGNOSIS 203
20.4 COMMON DIAGNOSTIC ERRORS AND HOW TO AVOID THEM 206

CHAPTER 21: ASSESSMENT TOOLS 211

21.1 OVERVIEW OF CLINICAL RATING SCALES 211
21.2 DIAGNOSTIC QUESTIONNAIRES AND SELF-REPORT TOOLS 214
21.3 FUNCTIONAL AND QUALITY OF LIFE ASSESSMENTS 217
21.4 CULTURAL CONSIDERATIONS IN ASSESSMENTS 219
21.5 INTERPRETATION OF ASSESSMENT RESULTS 221

CHAPTER 22: SUPPLEMENTARY ONLINE RESOURCES 225

ACCESS OUR VIRTUAL ASSISTANT 225

CONCLUSION 226

DISCLAIMER: The descriptions of DSM-5-TR disorders provided in this book are simplified and summarized to offer a quick reference and support learning. They are not intended to replace the complete DSM-5-TR text, which includes the full diagnostic criteria necessary for accurate clinical diagnosis. We strongly recommend using this book as a complementary tool alongside the official DSM-5-TR manual to reinforce your understanding and memory. Please refer to the DSM-5-TR for comprehensive diagnostic information and to ensure accuracy in clinical settings.

Section 1:
Introduction to DSM-5-TR and Clinical Diagnosis

Chapter 1: Introduction to DSM-5-TR

1.1 Key Updates in DSM-5-TR

Welcome to the first chapter of our journey into the world of DSM-5-TR and clinical diagnosis. As mental health professionals, it's crucial to stay informed about the latest developments and updates in our field, and the release of the DSM-5-TR marks a significant milestone. In this section, we'll dive into the key updates that have been introduced in this revised version of the Diagnostic and Statistical Manual of Mental Disorders.

One of the most notable changes in the DSM-5-TR is the inclusion of ICD-10-CM codes alongside the DSM-5 codes. This integration aims to facilitate a more seamless transition between the two coding systems and enhance communication among healthcare providers. By aligning the DSM-5-TR with the ICD-10-CM, clinicians can ensure more accurate documentation and improve the efficiency of the diagnostic process.

Another significant update in the DSM-5-TR is the refinement of diagnostic criteria for several disorders. These revisions are based on the latest research findings and clinical insights, aiming to enhance the precision and clarity of the diagnostic guidelines. For example, the criteria for Autism Spectrum Disorder have been updated to better capture the diverse presentations of the condition across the lifespan.

The DSM-5-TR also introduces a new disorder, Prolonged Grief Disorder, which recognizes the profound impact of persistent and impairing grief reactions. This addition reflects the growing understanding of the distinct nature of prolonged grief and its potential to significantly affect an individual's functioning.

Furthermore, the DSM-5-TR incorporates updated language and terminology to promote a more inclusive and culturally sensitive approach to mental health diagnosis. This includes revisions to the names of certain disorders and the use of gender-neutral pronouns throughout the manual.

It's important to note that while these updates aim to improve the diagnostic process, they also present an opportunity for mental health professionals to refine their skills and knowledge. Engaging with the DSM-5-TR updates through resources like this book will help you stay at the forefront of your field and provide the best possible care to your clients.

As we move through this chapter, we'll explore the purpose and application of the DSM-5-TR in clinical practice, equipping you with the tools and understanding needed to effectively utilize this essential resource. So, let's embrace the updates, dive into the details, and continue our journey towards diagnostic excellence.

1.2 Purpose of DSM-5-TR in Clinical Diagnosis

Now that we've explored the key updates in the DSM-5-TR, let's take a moment to reflect on the fundamental purpose of this diagnostic manual in clinical practice. As mental health professionals, we rely on the DSM-5-TR as a guiding light in our quest to accurately identify, understand, and treat mental health disorders. But what exactly makes this resource so invaluable?

At its core, the DSM-5-TR serves as a common language for mental health professionals across various disciplines. Whether you're a psychiatrist, psychologist, social worker, or counselor, the DSM-5-TR provides a standardized framework for describing and categorizing mental health conditions. By using a shared set of diagnostic criteria, we can ensure consistency and clarity in our communication with colleagues, clients, and healthcare systems.

But the DSM-5-TR is more than just a catalog of disorders; it's a tool that supports evidence-based practice. The diagnostic criteria outlined in the manual are grounded in extensive research and clinical expertise, reflecting the latest understanding of mental health conditions. By aligning our diagnostic process with the DSM-5-TR, we can have confidence that we're making informed decisions based on the best available evidence.

Moreover, the DSM-5-TR plays a crucial role in treatment planning and monitoring. Once a diagnosis is established using the criteria provided in the manual, clinicians can develop targeted interventions that address the specific symptoms and challenges faced by their clients. The DSM-5-TR also provides a framework for tracking treatment progress and adjusting interventions as needed, ensuring that clients receive the most effective care possible.

Beyond its clinical applications, the DSM-5-TR serves a broader purpose in advancing mental health research and policy. By providing a standardized language and criteria for mental health conditions, the manual enables researchers to conduct studies that deepen our understanding of these disorders and inform the development of new treatments. Additionally, the DSM-5-TR is often used as a reference point for mental health policy decisions, such as determining insurance coverage and allocating resources for mental health services.

As we navigate the complex landscape of mental health diagnosis, it's important to remember that the DSM-5-TR is a tool, not a rigid set of rules. While it provides a valuable framework, the manual should always be used in conjunction with clinical judgment, cultural considerations, and a person-centered approach. By combining the expertise of the DSM-5-TR with our own knowledge and skills, we can provide the highest quality of care to those we serve.

In the following chapters, we'll delve deeper into the practical applications of the DSM-5-TR, exploring how to effectively use this resource in our daily practice. Through interactive questions, real-world case studies, and step-by-step diagnostic guides, we'll equip you with the tools and confidence needed to harness the full potential of the DSM-5-TR in your clinical work. So, let's continue our journey together, armed with a clear understanding of the purpose and power of this essential diagnostic manual.

Chapter 2: How to Use This Book

2.1 Using Interactive Questions

Welcome to the second chapter of our journey through the DSM-5-TR Diagnostic Handbook. In this section, we'll explore one of the key features of this book: interactive questions. These questions are designed to engage you actively in the learning process, not merely as a means of testing your knowledge, but as a tool to foster a deeper, more practical understanding of the DSM-5-TR diagnostic criteria.

As mental health professionals, we know that diagnostic skills are best developed through hands-on experience and active engagement with the material. That's why the interactive questions in this book go beyond simple fact-checking. They are crafted to simulate real-world clinical scenarios, encouraging you to think as you would in an actual patient encounter.

Throughout Section 2, "*1000+ Interactive Questions to Test Your Knowledge*," you'll find a variety of question types designed to challenge and support your learning. Many questions are based on realistic clinical vignettes, presenting patient symptoms and histories, and asking you to identify the most likely diagnosis or differentiate between similar disorders. These scenario-based questions will help you sharpen your diagnostic acumen and prepare you for the complexities of real-world practice.

Other questions focus on diagnostic comparisons, helping you distinguish between disorders with overlapping symptoms. By engaging with these questions, you'll strengthen your differential diagnosis skills, a critical component of effective clinical decision-making. You'll also encounter questions that require you to choose the next step in a diagnostic process, simulating the step-by-step reasoning that underlies clinical assessment.

One of the unique features of the interactive questions in this book is the inclusion of detailed explanations for each answer. These explanations not only provide the correct response but also delve into the reasoning behind why other options are incorrect. By exploring these explanations, you'll gain a more nuanced understanding of the diagnostic criteria and the thought processes that guide clinical judgment.

In addition to the questions themselves, you'll find elements of self-assessment woven throughout the section. These reflective prompts invite you to consider which diagnostic criteria you found most challenging to remember, suggesting additional memorization exercises or practice opportunities. This self-directed learning approach empowers you to take an active role in your own professional development.

Some question sets are structured as scored quizzes, providing immediate feedback on your performance. These quizzes allow you to track your progress and identify areas where you may need further study or clarification. By engaging with these interactive features, you'll not only reinforce your knowledge but also build the confidence needed to apply the DSM-5-TR criteria effectively in your clinical work.

As we move through the interactive questions in Section 2, remember that the goal is not simply to memorize facts but to develop practical diagnostic skills. By immersing yourself in these questions and reflecting on the explanations provided, you'll cultivate the clinical reasoning abilities that are the hallmark of effective mental health practice.

So, let's dive into the world of interactive learning, embracing the challenges and opportunities presented by these carefully crafted questions. With each question you answer, each explanation you explore, you'll be taking another step towards mastering the art and science of diagnostic assessment using the DSM-5-TR. Onward!

2.2 Applying Real-World Clinical Cases

In the previous section, we explored the power of interactive questions in enhancing your understanding and application of the DSM-5-TR diagnostic criteria. Now, let's dive into another critical aspect of this book: real-world clinical cases. These carefully crafted case studies, found in Section 3, are designed to bridge the gap between theoretical knowledge and practical skills, preparing you for the challenges and complexities of real-life clinical scenarios.

As mental health professionals, we know that no two patients are exactly alike. Each individual brings a unique set of symptoms, experiences, and contextual factors that shape their presentation and inform our diagnostic approach. The real-world clinical cases in this book reflect this diversity, offering a wide range of scenarios that capture the nuances and intricacies of mental health assessment.

In Section 3, you'll find a rich tapestry of case studies, organized by diagnostic categories. From neurodevelopmental disorders to personality disorders, each chapter presents a series of cases that bring the DSM-5-TR criteria to life. These cases are not mere simplifications or stereotypes; they are grounded in the realities of clinical practice, reflecting the complex interplay of symptoms, comorbidities, and psychosocial factors that shape mental health presentations.

As you work through these cases, you'll have the opportunity to apply your diagnostic skills in a simulated clinical setting. Each case provides a detailed patient history, presenting symptoms, and relevant background information. Your task is to analyze this information, consider differential diagnoses, and arrive at a well-reasoned diagnostic conclusion based on the DSM-5-TR criteria.

But the learning process doesn't stop there. Each case is accompanied by a comprehensive discussion that explores the key diagnostic considerations, potential challenges, and best practices for assessment and treatment planning. These discussions are grounded in the latest research and clinical insights, providing a wealth of knowledge to inform your own practice.

One of the unique features of the real-world clinical cases in this book is the emphasis on cultural sensitivity and diversity. Mental health professionals must be attuned to the ways in which culture, ethnicity, race, gender, and other intersecting identities shape mental health experiences and expressions. The cases in this book reflect this diversity, challenging you to consider how cultural factors may influence diagnostic presentation and treatment approaches.

As you engage with these real-world cases, you'll not only sharpen your diagnostic skills but also develop a deeper appreciation for the complexity and individuality of each patient. You'll learn to approach assessment with a holistic, person-centered lens, considering not just the presence of symptoms but the unique context in which they occur.

The real-world clinical cases in this book are not meant to be prescriptive or exhaustive. Rather, they serve as a catalyst for your own clinical reasoning and professional growth. By grappling with these cases, discussing them with colleagues, and reflecting on your own approach, you'll cultivate the adaptability and critical thinking skills that are the hallmarks of effective mental health practice.

So, as we move into Section 3, embrace the challenge and opportunity presented by these real-world clinical cases. Immerse yourself in the rich narratives, apply your diagnostic acumen, and learn from the expert discussions provided. With each case you explore, you'll be one step closer to navigating the complexities of real-world mental health assessment with skill, sensitivity, and confidence.

2.3 Utilizing Step-by-Step Diagnostic Guides

As we continue our journey through the DSM-5-TR Diagnostic Handbook, we now turn our attention to a powerful tool designed to streamline and enhance your diagnostic process: step-by-step diagnostic guides. These guides, found in Section 4 of the book, provide a clear, systematic approach to applying the DSM-5-TR criteria in clinical practice, ensuring that you arrive at accurate and well-supported diagnostic conclusions.

Diagnosing mental health conditions is a complex and multifaceted process that requires careful consideration of a wide range of factors. From evaluating symptom presentations to ruling out differential diagnoses, the diagnostic journey can be challenging, even for experienced clinicians. The step-by-step diagnostic guides in this book are designed to provide a roadmap for navigating this complexity, breaking down the process into clear, manageable steps.

Each diagnostic guide follows a consistent structure, walking you through the key decision points and considerations involved in arriving at a specific diagnosis. The guides begin by outlining the essential diagnostic criteria for the disorder in question, providing a clear reference point for your assessment. From there, the guides lead you through a series of questions and prompts designed to help you gather and evaluate relevant clinical information.

One of the key features of these diagnostic guides is their emphasis on differential diagnosis. Mental health conditions often present with overlapping or similar symptoms, making it crucial to consider alternative explanations before arriving at a final diagnosis. The guides provide detailed information on common differential diagnoses, highlighting key distinguishing features and guiding you through the process of ruling out other conditions.

In addition to differential diagnosis, the step-by-step guides also address common diagnostic challenges and potential pitfalls. These may include considerations such as comorbidity, atypical presentations, or age-specific variations in symptom expression. By highlighting these potential challenges upfront, the guides help you anticipate and navigate the complexities of real-world diagnostic scenarios.

As you work through the step-by-step diagnostic guides, you'll find that they promote a thoughtful, systematic approach to assessment. Rather than simply providing a checklist of criteria, the guides encourage you to think critically about the information you gather, weighing evidence and considering alternative explanations. This process of active engagement with the diagnostic criteria helps to deepen your understanding of the conditions you are assessing and enhances your ability to make accurate, well-reasoned diagnoses.

One of the unique benefits of the step-by-step diagnostic guides in this book is their integration with the other learning tools provided. The guides often reference relevant interactive questions or real-world clinical cases, allowing you to apply your knowledge and skills in a variety of contexts. This integration creates a cohesive learning experience, reinforcing key concepts and promoting the transfer of knowledge to real-world practice.

As you utilize these step-by-step diagnostic guides, remember that they are intended to support, not replace, your clinical judgment. While the guides provide a valuable framework for assessment, they must always be used in conjunction with a holistic understanding of the individual you are evaluating. By combining the systematic approach of the guides with your own clinical expertise and patient-centered perspective, you'll be well-equipped to navigate even the most complex diagnostic challenges.

So, as we move into Section 4, embrace the clarity and structure provided by the step-by-step diagnostic guides. Let them serve as a compass, guiding you through the intricacies of the diagnostic process and empowering you to arrive at accurate, well-supported conclusions. With each guide you follow, you'll be refining your diagnostic skills and deepening your mastery of the DSM-5-TR criteria, preparing yourself for the realities of effective mental health practice.

2.4 Practical Application and Study Tips

As we conclude this chapter on how to use the DSM-5-TR Diagnostic Handbook, let's take a moment to consider some practical strategies for applying the knowledge and tools presented in this book. Learning the DSM-5-TR criteria and diagnostic processes is an ongoing journey, one that requires not just reading and memorization, but active engagement and real-world application.

One of the most effective ways to deepen your understanding of the DSM-5-TR is to make it a regular part of your clinical practice. As you encounter patients in your daily work, challenge yourself to apply the diagnostic criteria and step-by-step guides to their presenting concerns. Take note of any questions or uncertainties that arise, and use the interactive questions and real-world case studies in this book to explore these issues further.

Another key strategy is to engage in active, retrieval-based learning. Rather than simply reading through the diagnostic criteria or case studies, test your knowledge by actively recalling the information. Use flashcards, practice quizzes, or even discuss the criteria with colleagues to reinforce your understanding. The more actively you engage with the material, the more likely you are to retain and apply it effectively.

It's also important to approach your study of the DSM-5-TR with a growth mindset. Recognize that mastering diagnostic skills is a lifelong process, one that requires ongoing learning, reflection, and refinement. Embrace the challenges and uncertainties that arise in your practice, seeing them as opportunities for growth and development. When you encounter a complex case or a diagnostic dilemma, turn to the resources in this book and the expertise of your colleagues to deepen your understanding and expand your skills.

In addition to individual study and practice, consider forming a study group or joining a professional learning community focused on the DSM-5-TR. Collaborating with others allows you to benefit from diverse perspectives, share insights and challenges, and learn from the experiences of your peers. By engaging in collective learning and dialogue, you'll not only deepen your own understanding but also contribute to the growth and development of your professional community.

Finally, remember to approach your use of the DSM-5-TR with a person-centered, culturally sensitive lens. While the diagnostic criteria provide a valuable framework for assessment, they must always be applied in the context of the individual's unique experiences, cultural background, and social context. Take time to build rapport with your patients, gather a comprehensive history, and consider the ways in which their identity and environment may shape their mental health experiences. By combining the technical knowledge of the DSM-5-TR with a compassionate, individualized approach, you'll be well-equipped to provide effective, culturally responsive care.

As we move forward from this chapter, keep these practical strategies and tips in mind. The DSM-5-TR Diagnostic Handbook is a powerful tool, but its true value lies in the way you apply it in your daily practice. By engaging actively with the material, embracing ongoing learning, collaborating with others, and maintaining a person-centered approach, you'll be well on your way to mastering the art and science of diagnostic assessment.

So, let's continue our journey through the pages of this book, armed with a clear understanding of how to use its tools and insights to enhance your clinical practice. With each chapter, each question, each case study, you'll be refining your skills, expanding your knowledge, and deepening your ability to provide the highest quality care to those you serve. The path ahead is rich with opportunities for growth and discovery – let's embrace them together.

Chapter 3: **Diagnostic Tools and ICD-10-CM Codes**

3.1 Overview of Diagnostic Tools

Welcome to the third chapter of our exploration of the DSM-5-TR Diagnostic Handbook. In this section, we'll dive into the world of diagnostic tools, focusing on the resources and instruments that mental health professionals use to support and enhance the diagnostic process. These tools play a crucial role in our work, helping us to gather and organize clinical information, assess symptom severity, and make well-informed diagnostic decisions.

At the heart of the diagnostic toolkit is, of course, the DSM-5-TR itself. As we've explored in previous chapters, the DSM-5-TR provides a comprehensive framework for understanding and categorizing mental health conditions. Its diagnostic criteria and descriptive text serve as the foundation for our assessment process, guiding us in evaluating patients and arriving at accurate diagnoses.

But the DSM-5-TR is not the only tool at our disposal. In fact, there is a wide range of diagnostic instruments and resources available to support our work. These tools can be broadly categorized into several key types

1. Structured clinical interviews: These are standardized protocols for gathering clinical information, assessing symptoms, and determining whether diagnostic criteria are met. Examples include the Structured Clinical Interview for DSM-5 (SCID-5) and the Mini-International Neuropsychiatric Interview (MINI). Structured interviews provide a systematic, replicable approach to assessment, helping to ensure that all relevant information is gathered and that diagnoses are made consistently across patients and clinicians.

2. Rating scales and questionnaires: These are self-report or clinician-rated measures that assess the presence and severity of specific symptoms or conditions. Examples include the Beck Depression Inventory (BDI), the Generalized Anxiety Disorder 7-item scale (GAD-7), and the Patient Health Questionnaire-9 (PHQ-9). Rating scales provide a quantitative measure of symptom burden, allowing clinicians to track changes over time and assess treatment response.

3. Neuropsychological tests: These are specialized assessments that evaluate cognitive functioning, including memory, attention, executive function, and language skills. Examples include the Wechsler Adult Intelligence Scale (WAIS), the Trail Making Test, and the Wisconsin Card Sorting Test. Neuropsychological tests can help to identify cognitive deficits or strengths, informing diagnosis and treatment planning for conditions such as neurocognitive disorders or learning disabilities.

4. Personality assessments: These are tools designed to evaluate an individual's personality traits, patterns of behavior, and interpersonal style. Examples include the Minnesota Multiphasic Personality Inventory (MMPI), the Personality Assessment Inventory (PAI), and the Rorschach Inkblot Test. Personality assessments can provide valuable insights into an individual's underlying psychological makeup, informing diagnosis and treatment for conditions such as personality disorders.

5. Observational measures: These are tools that involve direct observation of an individual's behavior, either in a structured clinical setting or in their natural environment. Examples include the Autism Diagnostic Observation Schedule (ADOS) and the School Observation Scale. Observational measures can provide important information about how an individual functions in real-world contexts, complementing self-report and clinician-rated measures.

It's important to note that no single diagnostic tool is sufficient on its own. Rather, the most effective diagnostic approach involves using multiple tools and sources of information, integrating data from structured interviews, rating scales, observations, and other relevant sources. By using a multi-modal, comprehensive assessment strategy, we can develop a more complete understanding of an individual's symptoms, strengths, and challenges, leading to more accurate diagnoses and more effective treatment plans.

As we move through this chapter, we'll explore how these diagnostic tools intersect with the DSM-5-TR criteria and the ICD-10-CM coding system. We'll consider practical strategies for selecting and using diagnostic measures in clinical practice, and we'll discuss the important role that these tools play in treatment planning, progress monitoring, and insurance reimbursement.

So, let's dive in and explore the rich array of diagnostic tools at our disposal. By mastering these resources and integrating them effectively into our practice, we can enhance the precision, reliability, and clinical utility of our diagnostic assessments, ultimately leading to better outcomes for the individuals we serve.

3.2 DSM-5-TR and ICD-10-CM Criteria Mapping

As mental health professionals, we understand the critical importance of accurate diagnosis in guiding treatment planning and ensuring appropriate care for our patients. While the DSM-5-TR provides the foundational framework for our diagnostic assessments, it's essential to recognize the vital role that the International Classification of Diseases, 10th Revision, Clinical Modification (ICD-10-CM) plays in our work.

The ICD-10-CM is a comprehensive medical coding system used to classify and code diagnoses, symptoms, and procedures across all medical specialties, including mental health. Developed and maintained by the World Health Organization (WHO), the ICD-10-CM is used globally to track health statistics, monitor disease prevalence, and inform public health policy.

In the context of mental health diagnosis, the ICD-10-CM serves a crucial function in facilitating communication between clinicians, health systems, and insurance providers. When we assign an ICD-10-CM code to a patient's diagnosis, we're not just labeling their condition; we're providing a standardized, universally recognized descriptor that allows for consistent documentation, data analysis, and reimbursement.

One of the key features of the DSM-5-TR is its alignment with the ICD-10-CM coding system. Each diagnostic category and individual diagnosis in the DSM-5-TR is mapped to a corresponding ICD-10-CM code. This mapping ensures that the diagnostic terminology and criteria used in the DSM-5-TR are consistent with the ICD-10-CM, facilitating seamless communication and data exchange across healthcare systems.

To illustrate this mapping process, let's consider an example. A patient presents with symptoms of persistent, excessive worry, restlessness, fatigue, muscle tension, and sleep disturbance. Based on a comprehensive diagnostic assessment using DSM-5-TR criteria, the clinician determines that the patient meets the diagnostic threshold for Generalized Anxiety Disorder (GAD).

In the DSM-5-TR, GAD is listed under the category of Anxiety Disorders and is assigned the diagnostic code 300.02. This code corresponds directly to the ICD-10-CM code F41.1, which represents GAD. By assigning the F41.1 code to the patient's diagnosis, the clinician is not only documenting the specific condition but also facilitating communication with other healthcare providers and ensuring that the appropriate diagnostic information is captured for statistical and reimbursement purposes.

It's important to note that while the DSM-5-TR and ICD-10-CM are closely aligned, there are some differences in their organizational structures and diagnostic categories. For example, the ICD-10-CM includes certain conditions that are not present in the DSM-5-TR, such as Neurasthenia (F48.0) and Other Specified Behavioral and Emotional Disorders with Onset Usually Occurring in Childhood and Adolescence (F98.8).

Moreover, the ICD-10-CM is updated annually to reflect advances in medical knowledge and changes in diagnostic terminology. Mental health professionals must stay current with these updates to ensure that their diagnostic coding practices remain accurate and compliant with the latest guidelines.

As we navigate the complex landscape of mental health diagnosis, the DSM-5-TR and ICD-10-CM serve as essential tools in our diagnostic toolkit. By understanding the mapping between these two systems and utilizing them effectively in our practice, we can ensure that our patients receive the most appropriate, evidence-based care.

In the next section of this chapter, we'll explore the practical and insurance-related implications of ICD-10-CM coding, considering how these codes impact treatment authorization, reimbursement, and quality reporting. By mastering the intricacies of diagnostic coding, we can not only enhance the accuracy and consistency of our assessments but also advocate more effectively for our patients and support the long-term sustainability of our practices.

So, let's continue our journey into the world of diagnostic mapping, armed with a deeper understanding of the crucial intersection between the DSM-5-TR and ICD-10-CM. With each code we assign, each diagnosis we document, we're contributing to a larger system of knowledge and care, one that holds the power to transform lives and advance the field of mental health.

3.3 Practical and Insurance Use of ICD-10-CM Codes

As we've explored in the previous section, the ICD-10-CM coding system plays a vital role in the diagnostic process, facilitating communication and data exchange across healthcare settings. But the practical implications of ICD-10-CM codes extend far beyond the realm of clinical documentation. In fact, these codes are essential tools in navigating the complex world of insurance reimbursement and treatment authorization.

In the United States, the vast majority of mental health services are funded through insurance plans, whether private or public. These plans rely on ICD-10-CM codes to determine which services are medically necessary, which treatments are eligible for reimbursement, and how much providers will be paid for their services. As such, the accuracy and specificity of our diagnostic coding practices have a direct impact on our ability to secure appropriate care for our patients and maintain the financial viability of our practices.

When we assign an ICD-10-CM code to a patient's diagnosis, we're not just labeling their condition; we're providing a roadmap for their care. Insurance companies use these codes to determine whether a patient's symptoms and clinical presentation warrant coverage for specific treatments, such as psychotherapy, medication management, or hospitalization. By ensuring that our diagnostic codes accurately reflect the severity and nature of our patients' conditions, we can advocate more effectively for the services they need

Moreover, ICD-10-CM codes are used to track and analyze patterns of mental health care utilization and outcomes across populations. This data is critical for informing public health policy, allocating resources, and identifying areas for quality improvement. By using codes consistently and accurately, we contribute to a larger system of knowledge that can drive positive change in the mental health landscape.

But navigating the world of insurance reimbursement and ICD-10-CM coding can be complex and challenging. Insurance plans often have specific requirements for diagnostic documentation, such as the need to provide detailed clinical rationales or meet certain severity thresholds. Failure to meet these requirements can result in denied claims, delayed payments, or even allegations of fraud or abuse.

To ensure that our diagnostic coding practices are both clinically accurate and compliant with insurance requirements, it's essential to stay current with the latest guidelines and regulations. This may involve participating in continuing education courses, consulting with coding specialists, or utilizing coding reference tools and software

It's also important to understand the specific documentation requirements of the insurance plans we work with. This may involve familiarizing ourselves with their medical necessity criteria, using specific diagnostic templates or formats, or providing additional clinical information to support our coding decisions.

In addition to ensuring compliance, effective diagnostic coding can also help us to advocate for our patients and secure the resources they need. By using codes that accurately reflect the complexity and severity of our patients' conditions, we can justify the need for more intensive or specialized services, such as longer-term therapy or referrals to higher levels of care.

Ultimately, the practical and insurance-related implications of ICD-10-CM coding underscore the critical role that mental health professionals play in advocating for our patients and shaping the larger healthcare system. By mastering the intricacies of diagnostic coding and using it effectively in our practice, we can ensure that our patients receive the care they need while also contributing to a more equitable, evidence-based mental health landscape.

As we conclude this chapter on diagnostic tools and ICD-10-CM codes, let's reflect on the power and responsibility we hold as mental health professionals. With each diagnosis we make, each code we assign, we have the opportunity to make a profound difference in the lives of our patients and the larger mental health community. By approaching this work with diligence, integrity, and a commitment to excellence, we can harness the power of diagnostic tools to drive meaningful, lasting change.

So, let's move forward with confidence and purpose, armed with the knowledge and skills we need to navigate the complex world of mental health diagnosis. Together, we can build a future in which every individual has access to the care and support they need to thrive.

Chapter 4: **Neurodevelopmental Disorders**

4.1 ADHD

1. A 9-year-old boy presents with symptoms including frequent fidgeting, difficulty staying seated in the classroom, and excessive talking. These behaviors have been present for 4 months and are causing significant problems at school, but his behavior at home is described as "normal." Which of the following is the most appropriate diagnostic consideration?
   A) ADHD, Combined Presentation
   B) ADHD, Predominantly Hyperactive Presentation
   C) The duration is insufficient for an ADHD diagnosis
   D) The symptoms do not meet cross-setting criteria

2. A 7-year-old child presents with difficulty maintaining attention, frequently making careless mistakes, and appearing not to listen when spoken to directly. These symptoms emerged shortly after a major family relocation. Which of the following should be considered first in the differential diagnosis?
   A) ADHD, Predominantly Inattentive Presentation
   B) Adjustment Disorder
   C) Specific Learning Disorder
   D) Anxiety Disorder

3. After identifying multiple ADHD symptoms in an adult patient, what is the most crucial next step in the diagnostic process?

A) Immediately initiate stimulant medication
B) Obtain developmental history and evidence of childhood onset
C) Order neuropsychological testing
D) Start behavioral therapy

4. A 10-year-old meets full criteria for ADHD, Combined Presentation, with significant impairment in both school and home settings. Which of the following is the most appropriate initial treatment approach according to current guidelines?
   A) Behavioral therapy alone
   B) FDA-approved medication alone
   C) Combined medication and behavioral therapy
   D) Watchful waiting with environmental modifications

5. Which of the following would be most suggestive that a child's inattentive symptoms might NOT be due to ADHD?
   A) Symptoms are worse in the morning
   B) Symptoms fluctuate significantly from day to day
   C) Symptoms appear only in challenging academic subjects
   D) Symptoms improve with structure and routine

4.2 Autism Spectrum Disorder

6. A 3-year-old child demonstrates no pretend play, does not respond to his name, has not developed any spoken language, and engages in repetitive hand-flapping. He shows no interest in other children and prefers to play alone. Parents report these behaviors have been present since age 18 months. Which is the most appropriate diagnostic consideration?

   A) Early-onset Schizophrenia

   B) Language Development Disorder

   C) Autism Spectrum Disorder

   D) Social Communication Disorder

7. During a clinical evaluation, a 5-year-old girl makes good eye contact but insists on organizing her toys in precise lines, becomes extremely distressed when routines change, and speaks in an unusually formal manner for her age. She has a few friends but struggles with reciprocal conversation. Which feature most strongly supports an ASD diagnosis?

   A) The presence of good eye contact

   B) The formal speech patterns

   C) The rigid adherence to routines

   D) The difficulty with reciprocal conversation

8. A 4-year-old demonstrates appropriate language development and intellectual ability but shows intense preoccupation with train schedules, becomes highly distressed with minor changes in routine, and has difficulty understanding social cues. What should be the next step in the diagnostic process?

   A) Rule out Obsessive-Compulsive Disorder

   B) Conduct comprehensive autism evaluation

   C) Start speech therapy immediately

   D) Diagnose Social Communication Disorder

9. Parents of a 2-year-old are concerned because their child has not developed any words, shows no interest in other children, and does not point to objects of interest. The pediatrician is considering ASD. Which of the following is the most appropriate next step?

   A) Wait and see approach until age 3

   B) Immediate referral for comprehensive ASD evaluation

   C) Start speech therapy only

   D) Prescribe antipsychotic medication

10. A 6-year-old child was diagnosed with ASD at age 3. She has made significant progress with interventions but still shows some social communication difficulties and restricted interests. Her parents report she no longer meets full criteria for ASD. Which is the most appropriate diagnostic conclusion?

   A) Remove the ASD diagnosis completely

   B) Maintain the ASD diagnosis with current severity specification

   C) Change diagnosis to Social Communication Disorder

   D) Change diagnosis to Unspecified Neurodevelopmental Disorder

4.3 Intellectual Disabilities

11. A 6-year-old child is referred for evaluation due to significant academic difficulties. Testing reveals an IQ of 65, with significant deficits in adaptive functioning across multiple domains, including self-care, social skills, and academic performance. Parents report developmental delays were noticed since age 2. Which is the most appropriate diagnosis?

    A) Specific Learning Disorder

    B) Mild Intellectual Disability

    C) Global Developmental Delay

    D) Borderline Intellectual Functioning

12. During the assessment of a 7-year-old with suspected intellectual disability, which of the following adaptive functioning deficits would be MOST significant in supporting the diagnosis?

    A) Difficulty with advanced mathematical calculations

    B) Poor handwriting skills

    C) Inability to handle age-appropriate self-care tasks

    D) Limited participation in team sports

13. A 4-year-old child shows significant developmental delays. Which sequence of diagnostic steps is most appropriate?

    A) IQ testing immediately followed by placement in special education

    B) Comprehensive medical evaluation, then adaptive functioning assessment, then cognitive testing

    C) Start behavioral therapy, then assess progress, then consider testing

    D) Wait until school age for formal assessment

14. Parents of a child diagnosed with moderate intellectual disability (IQ 45) ask about prognosis and treatment. Which statement best represents current evidence-based guidance?

    A) The child will never be able to live independently

    B) With proper support, improvements in adaptive functioning are possible

    C) Medication is the primary treatment approach

D) Academic achievement is impossible

15. A teenager with mild intellectual disability (IQ 65) is being evaluated for depression. Which of the following approaches is most appropriate for diagnostic assessment?

A) Rely solely on parent/caregiver report

B) Use standard adult depression criteria

C) Modify assessment approach based on developmental level

D) Assume symptoms are due to intellectual disability

4.4 Communication Disorders

16. A 4-year-old child speaks in simple phrases, has difficulty being understood by strangers, makes frequent sound substitutions, and demonstrates age-appropriate comprehension. Development history shows no other concerns. Which diagnosis is most likely?

A) Autism Spectrum Disorder

B) Speech Sound Disorder

C) Language Disorder

D) Social Communication Disorder

17. A 3-year-old who previously spoke in 2-3 word phrases has shown a significant decline in speech production over the past 2 months, though comprehension remains intact. Which diagnostic step should be prioritized?

A) Start speech therapy immediately

B) Diagnose Childhood Apraxia of Speech

C) Conduct urgent medical evaluation

D) Wait and monitor for 6 months

18. An 8-year-old student has normal articulation and vocabulary but consistently struggles with understanding complex sentences, following multi-step directions, and organizing narrative discourse. Which diagnosis should be considered first?

A) Social Communication Disorder

B) Specific Learning Disorder

C) Language Disorder

D) Attention-Deficit/Hyperactivity Disorder

19. A 5-year-old child stutters severely, showing frequent sound prolongations and blocks. The parents ask about the best timing for intervention. Which response is most appropriate based on current evidence?

A) Wait until age 7 when stuttering typically resolves

B) Begin immediate intervention due to age and severity

C) Focus only on parent counseling for now

D) Treat only if the child shows anxiety

20. A 6-year-old bilingual child is referred for speech evaluation. He shows similar language difficulties in both languages, with poor grammar and limited vocabulary. Which statement is most accurate regarding diagnosis?

A) Assessment in English only is sufficient

B) Difficulties must be present in both languages for diagnosis

C) Wait for dominance in one language before assessment

D) Language disorder can't be diagnosed in bilingual children

4.5 Specific Learning Disorders

21. A 9-year-old student with average intelligence shows persistent difficulty with reading accuracy and fluency despite adequate instruction and intervention. Their reading performance is significantly below grade level, impacting academic achievement. Which diagnostic consideration is most appropriate?

    A) Specific Learning Disorder with impairment in reading

    B) Intellectual Disability

    C) Attention-Deficit/Hyperactivity Disorder

    D) Language Disorder

22. During evaluation of a 7-year-old with possible learning difficulties, which of the following findings would be MOST important in establishing a diagnosis of Specific Learning Disorder?

    A) Parent report of homework struggles

    B) Below average performance on standardized achievement tests

    C) Academic skills substantially below expectations for age plus adequate intervention response data

    D) Teacher concern about classroom behavior

23. A third-grade student shows significant difficulty with mathematical calculation and problem-solving, but reads and writes at grade level. IQ testing indicates average intelligence. What is the next appropriate step in the diagnostic process?

    A) Begin interventions without formal testing

    B) Conduct comprehensive psychoeducational evaluation

    C) Wait another year to see if skills improve

    D) Focus solely on math tutoring

24. A student diagnosed with Specific Learning Disorder with impairment in reading shows adequate decoding skills but significant difficulty with reading comprehension. Which specifier is most appropriate?

A) Dyslexia

B) Impairment in reading comprehension

C) Mixed reading disorder

D) Impairment in basic reading skills

25. A 10-year-old presents with difficulty in writing, including poor spelling, grammar errors, and problems with written expression. Academic history shows persistent struggles despite regular instruction. What additional information is MOST crucial for diagnosis?

A) Family history of learning disorders

B) Results of vision screening

C) Evidence that difficulties exceed age-appropriate variations

D) Social skills assessment

4.6 Motor Disorders

26. A 5-year-old child shows significant difficulty with age-appropriate motor skills, including buttoning clothes, using scissors, and catching a ball. Intelligence and social development are normal. Which preliminary diagnosis should be considered?

A) Autism Spectrum Disorder

B) Developmental Coordination Disorder

C) Stereotypic Movement Disorder

D) ADHD, predominantly hyperactive type

27. During evaluation of a child with possible Developmental Coordination Disorder, which clinical finding would be MOST important in establishing the diagnosis?

A) Poor handwriting in isolation

B) Motor skills substantially below age expectations affecting daily activities

C) Parent report of clumsiness

D) Poor performance in physical education class

28. A 7-year-old displays repetitive hand flapping and body rocking that interfere with normal activities and have caused mild self-injury. These movements increase with stress. No developmental delays are noted. Which diagnosis is most appropriate?

A) Autism Spectrum Disorder

B) Tourette's Disorder

C) Stereotypic Movement Disorder

D) Obsessive-Compulsive Disorder

29. A 6-year-old presents with sudden onset of motor and vocal tics including eye blinking and throat clearing. What is the most appropriate initial clinical approach?

A) Immediate initiation of antipsychotic medication

B) Monitor symptoms for duration and impact

C) Diagnose Tourette's Disorder

D) Refer for immediate neurological evaluation

30. A 4-year-old shows delayed motor development and hypotonia. Before diagnosing a motor disorder, which assessment is MOST crucial?

A) Occupational therapy evaluation

B) Neurological examination and medical workup

C) Psychological assessment

D) Educational evaluation

Chapter 5: Schizophrenia Spectrum and Other Psychotic Disorders

5.1 Schizophrenia

1. A 22-year-old male presents with auditory hallucinations, paranoid delusions, and social withdrawal for 8 months. His academic performance has declined significantly, and he has stopped attending college. No mood episodes are present. Which diagnosis is most appropriate?

   A) Brief Psychotic Disorder

   B) Schizophreniform Disorder

   C) Schizophrenia

   D) Major Depressive Disorder with Psychotic Features

2. During the evaluation of a patient with suspected schizophrenia, which combination of symptoms would be MOST supportive of the diagnosis?

   A) Depression and anxiety

   B) Delusions and disorganized speech

   C) Memory problems and confusion

   D) Mood swings and irritability

3. A patient diagnosed with schizophrenia has been experiencing predominantly negative symptoms (flat affect, avolition, alogia). Which of the following treatment approaches should be prioritized?

   A) High-dose antipsychotic medication

   B) Psychosocial rehabilitation and supported employment

   C) Electroconvulsive therapy

   D) Benzodiazepines

4. A 19-year-old develops psychotic symptoms two weeks after starting college. Which sequence of diagnostic steps is most appropriate?

   A) Start antipsychotics and monitor response

   B) Medical workup, toxicology screen, then psychological assessment

   C) Wait for symptoms to persist for 6 months

   D) Immediate hospitalization without further evaluation

5. A patient with schizophrenia shows good response to treatment but expresses concern about relapse. Which factor is MOST important in preventing relapse?

   A) Regular blood tests

   B) Medication adherence and continued psychosocial support

   C) Monthly psychiatrist visits

   D) Family therapy alone

5.2 Schizoaffective Disorder

6. A 25-year-old presents with delusions, hallucinations, and a major depressive episode. Their history reveals psychotic symptoms persisting for several weeks after mood symptoms have resolved. Which diagnosis is most appropriate?

   A) Major Depressive Disorder with psychotic features

   B) Schizoaffective Disorder, depressive type

   C) Schizophrenia with comorbid depression

   D) Bipolar Disorder with psychotic features

7. In differentiating between Schizoaffective Disorder and Schizophrenia with comorbid mood symptoms, which clinical feature is MOST decisive?

   A) Severity of psychotic symptoms

   B) Duration of mood symptoms relative to total illness duration

   C) Age of onset

   D) Family history of mental illness

8. A patient with suspected Schizoaffective Disorder shows both manic and depressive episodes along with persistent delusions. What additional information is MOST critical for accurate diagnosis?

   A) Response to antipsychotic medication

   B) Presence of psychotic symptoms during mood-free periods

   C) Sleep patterns during mood episodes

   D) Cognitive functioning assessment

9. Which treatment approach is most appropriate for a newly diagnosed patient with Schizoaffective Disorder, bipolar type?

   A) Antipsychotic medication alone

   B) Mood stabilizer alone

   C) Combined mood stabilizer and antipsychotic medication

   D) Antidepressant monotherapy

10. A patient diagnosed with Schizoaffective Disorder has been stable on medication for one year but continues to have mild residual symptoms. Which outcome measure is MOST important in assessing recovery?

    A) Complete resolution of all symptoms

    B) Level of social and occupational functioning

    C) Number of hospitalizations

    D) Medication dose requirements

5.3 Delusional Disorder

11. A 45-year-old professional presents with a 2-year history of believing their spouse is unfaithful, despite no evidence. They function well at work and have no other psychotic symptoms. Which diagnosis is most appropriate?

    A) Delusional Disorder, jealous type

    B) Schizophrenia

    C) Obsessive-Compulsive Disorder

    D) Major Depressive Disorder with psychotic features

12. Which clinical feature is MOST characteristic of Delusional Disorder when comparing it to other psychotic disorders?

    A) Presence of hallucinations

    B) Intact occupational functioning outside delusional content

    C) Multiple types of delusions

    D) Disorganized behavior

13. A patient presents with fixed beliefs about having a serious illness despite multiple normal medical evaluations. Apart from health anxiety, functioning is preserved. What is the next most appropriate diagnostic step?

    A) Order additional medical tests

    B) Evaluate for Delusional Disorder, somatic type

    C) Refer to an infectious disease specialist

    D) Start high-dose antipsychotics immediately

14. In treating a patient with Delusional Disorder, which therapeutic approach is most appropriate initially?

    A) Directly challenging the delusions

    B) Building therapeutic alliance while avoiding direct confrontation

    C) Intensive cognitive behavioral therapy

    D) Immediate high-dose antipsychotic medication

15. A patient with Delusional Disorder believes the government is monitoring them through electronic devices. Which aspect of assessment is MOST important for risk evaluation?

    A) Family history of psychosis

    B) Presence of hallucinations

    C) Potential for acting on delusions

    D) Duration of symptoms

5.4 Brief Psychotic Disorder

16. A 28-year-old woman develops sudden onset of delusions and hallucinations three days after giving birth. No previous psychiatric history. Symptoms have lasted 5 days. Which diagnosis is most appropriate?

    A) Postpartum Depression

    B) Brief Psychotic Disorder with postpartum onset

    C) Schizophrenia

    D) Bipolar Disorder with psychotic features

17. Which duration criterion is essential for diagnosing Brief Psychotic Disorder according to DSM-5-TR?

    A) Symptoms lasting at least 6 months

    B) Symptoms lasting 1-6 months

    C) Symptoms lasting 1 day to 1 month

    D) Symptoms lasting less than 1 day

18. A 35-year-old develops psychotic symptoms following a severe earthquake disaster. Which feature is MOST important in determining the specifier "with marked stressor"?

    A) Severity of psychotic symptoms

    B) Temporal relationship between stressor and onset

    C) Previous psychiatric history

    D) Family history of psychosis

19. In evaluating a possible Brief Psychotic Disorder, which clinical consideration is MOST critical for initial management?

    A) Family psychiatric history

    B) Detailed childhood history

    C) Rule out medical/substance-induced causes

    D) Genetic testing

20. A patient diagnosed with Brief Psychotic Disorder has complete symptom resolution after 3 weeks. What is the most appropriate follow-up plan?

    A) Discontinue all treatment immediately

    B) Maintain antipsychotics indefinitely

    C) Monitor for recurrence while gradually reducing treatment

    D) Start long-term psychotherapy

5.5 Catatonia

21. A patient presents with mutism, posturing, and waxy flexibility during a major depressive episode. What is the most appropriate diagnostic formulation?

    A) Major Depressive Disorder with catatonic features

    B) Schizophrenia, catatonic type

    C) Catatonia due to medical condition

    D) Brief Psychotic Disorder

22. Which combination of symptoms is MOST specific for diagnosing catatonia according to DSM-5-TR?

    A) Depression and anxiety

    B) Stupor and waxy flexibility

    C) Confusion and disorientation

    D) Delusions and hallucinations

23. A patient develops sudden onset of catatonic symptoms. Which initial assessment is MOST crucial?

    A) Psychiatric history

    B) Comprehensive medical workup including vital signs

    C) Family history of mental illness

    D) Childhood developmental history

24. In treating a patient with catatonia, which intervention should typically be initiated first?

A) Electroconvulsive therapy

B) Trial of benzodiazepines

C) Antipsychotic medications

D) Supportive psychotherapy

25. A patient with catatonia shows signs of autonomic instability and hyperthermia. Which complication should be urgently ruled out?

A) Delirium

B) Major Depression

C) Malignant Catatonia

D) Conversion Disorder

Chapter 6: **Bipolar and Related Disorders**

6.1 Bipolar I Disorder

1. A 23-year-old presents with a first episode of decreased need for sleep, pressured speech, grandiose ideas, and risky financial behavior lasting 2 weeks. The patient has a history of depression. Which diagnosis is most appropriate?

   A) Bipolar II Disorder

   B) Bipolar I Disorder

   C) Substance-Induced Mood Disorder

   D) Major Depressive Disorder with agitation

2. During assessment of a possible manic episode, which combination of symptoms is MOST definitive for diagnosis according to DSM-5-TR?

   A) Irritability and anxiety

   B) Decreased need for sleep and grandiosity

   C) Racing thoughts and depression

   D) Increased appetite and insomnia

3. A patient with Bipolar I Disorder presents with acute mania including psychotic features. Which treatment sequence is most appropriate?

   A) Start antidepressant immediately

   B) Begin mood stabilizer and monitor weekly

   C) Initiate acute antimanic medication and consider hospitalization

   D) Prescribe benzodiazepines alone

4. In evaluating long-term treatment response for Bipolar I Disorder, which outcome measure is MOST important?

   A) Resolution of current episode only

   B) Prevention of both manic and depressive episodes

   C) Social functioning only

   D) Medication side effects only

5. A patient with well-controlled Bipolar I Disorder becomes pregnant. Which clinical consideration is MOST critical?

   A) Immediate discontinuation of all medications

   B) Risk-benefit analysis of medication continuation

   C) Switch to antidepressant monotherapy

   D) Wait until delivery to adjust treatment

6.2 Bipolar II Disorder

6. A patient presents with recurrent major depressive episodes and a history of periods of increased productivity, decreased need for sleep, and elevated mood lasting 3 days without significant impairment. Which diagnosis is most appropriate?

   A) Major Depressive Disorder

   B) Bipolar I Disorder

   C) Bipolar II Disorder

   D) Cyclothymic Disorder

7. In differentiating between Bipolar I and Bipolar II Disorder, which clinical feature is MOST decisive?

   A) Age of onset

   B) Presence of psychotic features

   C) Severity of depressive episodes

   D) Severity and consequences of elevated mood episodes

8. A patient with Bipolar II Disorder reports increased energy, activity, and mild euphoria for 2 days. Which assessment focus is MOST important?

   A) Previous depressive episodes

   B) Whether criteria for hypomania are met

   C) Family history of bipolar disorder

   D) Current medication compliance

9. Which treatment approach is most appropriate for acute management of Bipolar II Depression?

   A) Antidepressant monotherapy

   B) Mood stabilizer with possible careful antidepressant addition

   C) High-dose antipsychotics

   D) Benzodiazepines alone

10. A patient with Bipolar II Disorder reports "feeling better than ever" with increased goal-directed activity. Which monitoring focus is most crucial?

   A) Sleep patterns and activity level

   B) Appetite changes only

   C) Memory function

   D) Physical health only

6.3 Cyclothymic Disorder

11. A patient reports a 2-year history of frequent mood fluctuations between mild depression and elevated mood, never meeting full criteria for major depression or mania/hypomania. Which diagnosis is most appropriate?

   A) Bipolar I Disorder

   B) Bipolar II Disorder

   C) Cyclothymic Disorder

   D) Persistent Depressive Disorder

12. Which duration criterion must be met for diagnosing Cyclothymic Disorder in adults according to DSM-5-TR?

A) At least 6 months of symptoms

B) At least 1 year of symptoms

C) At least 2 years of symptoms

D) At least 3 years of symptoms

13. A teenager presents with alternating periods of mild elation and depressive symptoms. During evaluation for Cyclothymic Disorder, which clinical feature is MOST important to assess?

A) Family history of mood disorders

B) Duration and severity of mood episodes

C) School performance only

D) Sleep patterns only

14. What is the most appropriate initial treatment approach for a newly diagnosed patient with Cyclothymic Disorder?

A) High-dose antipsychotics

B) Psychoeducation and mood monitoring

C) Immediate antidepressant therapy

D) Intensive psychoanalysis

15. Which factor is MOST important in differentiating Cyclothymic Disorder from normal mood variation?

A) Number of episodes per year

B) Presence of psychotic features

C) Chronicity and functional impact

D) Age of onset

6.4 Substance/Medication-Induced Bipolar Disorder

16. A patient develops manic symptoms two days after starting corticosteroid treatment for an autoimmune condition. No previous psychiatric history. Which diagnosis is most appropriate?

    A) Bipolar I Disorder

    B) Substance/Medication-Induced Bipolar Disorder

    C) Steroid-Induced Psychosis

    D) Delirium

17. Which temporal relationship is MOST important in diagnosing Substance/Medication-Induced Bipolar Disorder?

    A) Symptoms present for at least 6 months

    B) Symptoms developing during or soon after substance use/medication

    C) Symptoms lasting after substance discontinuation

    D) Symptoms present before substance use

18. A patient presents with manic symptoms while using cocaine. Which assessment approach is MOST appropriate for accurate diagnosis?

    A) Immediate initiation of mood stabilizers

    B) Wait for 2 weeks of sobriety before assessment

    C) Evaluate onset, course, and previous history

    D) Focus only on current symptoms

19. Which intervention should be prioritized in managing substance-induced manic symptoms?

    A) Continue current medications unchanged

    B) Address the underlying substance use/medication issue

    C) Start long-term antipsychotic treatment

    D) Begin intensive psychotherapy

20. A patient develops hypomanic symptoms after starting an antidepressant. Which management strategy is most appropriate?

A) Continue antidepressant at current dose

B) Gradually reduce or discontinue antidepressant

C) Add a second antidepressant

D) Start lithium immediately

6.5 Other Specified Bipolar Disorders

21. A patient experiences hypomanic episodes lasting only 2-3 days, with significant functional impact and a history of major depression. Which diagnosis best fits this presentation?

A) Bipolar II Disorder

B) Other Specified Bipolar Disorder

C) Cyclothymic Disorder

D) Unspecified Mood Disorder

22. Which clinical presentation would most appropriately be classified as Other Specified Bipolar Disorder?

A) Full criteria manic episode lasting 7 days

B) Hypomanic episodes without history of depression

C) Major depressive episode with some mixed features

D) Classic bipolar I presentation

23. A patient has clear hypomanic symptoms but episodes last only 2 days. During evaluation, which factor is MOST important to assess?

A) Family history only

B) Impact on functioning and distress level

C) Childhood trauma history

D) Current medications only

24. In treating a patient with Other Specified Bipolar Disorder with short-duration hypomania, which approach is most appropriate?

    A) Observation only without intervention

    B) Same approach as Bipolar II Disorder

    C) Antidepressant monotherapy

    D) High-dose antipsychotics

25. When monitoring a patient with Other Specified Bipolar Disorder, which aspect is MOST important for ongoing assessment?

    A) Only tracking full manic episodes

    B) Potential evolution into other bipolar disorders

    C) Physical health only

    D) Social relationships only

Chapter 7: Depressive Disorders

7.1 Major Depressive Disorder

1. A 35-year-old presents with depressed mood, anhedonia, insomnia, fatigue, and feelings of worthlessness for 6 weeks, causing significant work impairment. What additional information is MOST crucial for diagnosis?

   A) Family history of depression

   B) History of manic/hypomanic episodes

   C) Childhood trauma history

   D) Previous medication trials

2. During assessment of Major Depressive Disorder, a patient reports passive suicidal thoughts. Which aspect of suicide risk assessment should be prioritized?

   A) Family history of suicide

   B) Specific plan and intent

   C) Past suicide attempts

   D) Current living situation

3. A patient with Major Depressive Disorder shows minimal response after 6 weeks on an SSRI at adequate dose. Which treatment approach is most appropriate?

   A) Immediately switch to a different antidepressant class

   B) Evaluate adherence, optimize dose, consider augmentation

   C) Add a second SSRI

   D) Discontinue medication and switch to psychotherapy only

4. A pregnant patient is diagnosed with moderate to severe MDD. Which treatment consideration is MOST important?

A) Avoid all medications during pregnancy

B) Risk-benefit analysis of treatment options including medication

C) Use psychotherapy only regardless of severity

D) Wait until after delivery to start treatment

5. After achieving remission from MDD, what is the most appropriate duration for continuation phase treatment?

A) 1-2 months

B) 4-6 months

C) At least 6-12 months

D) 2 weeks

7.2 Persistent Depressive Disorder (Dysthymia)

6. A patient reports chronic low mood, poor appetite, and low self-esteem for the past 3 years, with symptoms present most days. No major depressive episodes. Which diagnosis is most appropriate?

A) Major Depressive Disorder

B) Persistent Depressive Disorder

C) Adjustment Disorder

D) Cyclothymic Disorder

7. Which duration criterion must be met for diagnosing Persistent Depressive Disorder in adults according to DSM-5-TR?

A) At least 6 months

B) At least 1 year

C) At least 2 years

D) At least 3 years

8. A patient with Persistent Depressive Disorder develops symptoms meeting criteria for Major Depression. Which diagnostic specifier is most appropriate?

A) Mixed Anxiety Depression

B) With Seasonal Pattern

C) With Persistent Major Depressive Episode ("Double Depression")

D) With Melancholic Features

9. In treating Persistent Depressive Disorder, which initial approach has the strongest evidence base?

A) Psychotherapy alone

B) Combined psychotherapy and pharmacotherapy

C) Medication alone

D) Alternative therapies only

10. Which factor is MOST important in differentiating Persistent Depressive Disorder from chronic Major Depressive Disorder?

A) Number of symptoms

B) Severity of symptoms

C) Impact on functioning

D) Type of symptoms

7.3 Disruptive Mood Dysregulation Disorder

11. A 9-year-old child presents with severe, recurrent temper outbursts (3-4 times weekly) and persistently irritable mood between outbursts for over one year. Symptoms occur at home and school. Which diagnosis is most appropriate?

A) Oppositional Defiant Disorder

B) Disruptive Mood Dysregulation Disorder

C) Intermittent Explosive Disorder

D) Pediatric Bipolar Disorder

12. What is the age requirement for diagnosing Disruptive Mood Dysregulation Disorder according to DSM-5-TR?

    A) Symptoms must begin before age 6

    B) Symptoms must begin before age 10

    C) Diagnosis must be made before age 18

    D) Diagnosis must be made before age 12

13. A child with frequent aggressive outbursts is being evaluated for DMDD. Which additional clinical feature is MOST important to establish the diagnosis?

    A) Family history of mood disorders

    B) Persistent negative mood between outbursts

    C) Academic performance

    D) Social skills assessment

14. What is the most appropriate initial treatment approach for a newly diagnosed case of DMDD?

    A) Immediate mood stabilizer medication

    B) Parent training and behavioral intervention

    C) Antipsychotic medication

    D) Intensive individual psychotherapy only

15. In differentiating DMDD from pediatric bipolar disorder, which feature is MOST decisive?

    A) Severity of aggression

    B) Pattern of mood disturbance (persistent vs. episodic)

    C) Age of onset

    D) Gender of the child

7.4 Premenstrual Dysphoric Disorder

16. A woman reports severe mood symptoms (irritability, anxiety, depression) and physical symptoms occurring only during the week before menses for the past year, with significant functional impairment. Which diagnosis is most appropriate?

    A) Major Depressive Disorder

    B) Premenstrual Dysphoric Disorder

    C) Premenstrual Syndrome

    D) Generalized Anxiety Disorder

17. According to DSM-5-TR, how many cycles of prospective daily symptom ratings are required to confirm a PMDD diagnosis?

    A) At least 1 cycle

    B) At least 2 consecutive cycles

    C) At least 3 cycles

    D) At least 6 cycles

18. Which symptom pattern is MOST characteristic of PMDD?

    A) Constant symptoms throughout the month

    B) Symptoms only during menstruation

    C) Symptoms in luteal phase with premenstrual worsening and post-menstrual resolution

    D) Random symptom occurrence unrelated to menstrual cycle

19. In treating PMDD, which first-line treatment approach has the strongest evidence base?

    A) Herbal supplements only

    B) SSRIs (continuous or luteal phase)

    C) Psychotherapy alone

    D) Hormonal contraception only

20. A patient with suspected PMDD reports similar symptoms throughout her cycle. Which diagnostic step is most appropriate?

A) Increase the antidepressant dose

B) Re-evaluate for other mood disorders

C) Add anxiety medication

D) Dismiss the possibility of PMDD

7.5 Substance/Medication-Induced Depressive Disorder

21. A patient develops significant depressive symptoms two weeks after starting interferon treatment for hepatitis C. No prior psychiatric history. Which diagnosis is most appropriate?

A) Major Depressive Disorder

B) Substance/Medication-Induced Depressive Disorder

C) Adjustment Disorder

D) Organic Mood Disorder

22. In diagnosing Substance/Medication-Induced Depressive Disorder, which temporal relationship is MOST important to establish?

A) Depression present before substance use

B) Depression developing during or soon after substance use/medication

C) Depression persisting for 6 months

D) Depression occurring only during withdrawal

23. A patient presents with depressive symptoms while actively using alcohol. Which diagnostic approach is most appropriate?

A) Immediately diagnose Major Depression

B) Wait 4 weeks after sobriety before diagnosing

C) Start antidepressants immediately

D) Assess onset relative to substance use and obtain historical data

24. Which management strategy should be prioritized for medication-induced depression?

A) Add a second antidepressant

B) Consult with prescribing physician about medication adjustment

C) Start long-term psychotherapy

D) Ignore the medication's role

25. A patient develops depression while taking beta-blockers for hypertension. Which factor is MOST important in treatment planning?

A) Family history of depression

B) Risk-benefit analysis of continuing current medication

C) Past psychiatric history only

D) Patient's age

Chapter 8: **Anxiety Disorders**

8.1 Generalized Anxiety Disorder

1. A 32-year-old presents with excessive worry about multiple life areas (work, finances, health, family) for the past 8 months, along with restlessness, difficulty concentrating, and muscle tension. The worries interfere with daily functioning. What is the most appropriate diagnosis?

   A) Adjustment Disorder with Anxiety

   B) Generalized Anxiety Disorder

   C) Social Anxiety Disorder

   D) Obsessive-Compulsive Disorder

2. A patient meets criteria for GAD but also reports panic attacks. Which clinical feature is MOST important in determining if a separate panic disorder diagnosis is warranted?

   A) Frequency of panic attacks

   B) Whether panic attacks are expected vs. unexpected

   C) Severity of physical symptoms

   D) Time of day attacks occur

3. During evaluation of suspected GAD, which aspect should be prioritized to establish accurate diagnosis?

   A) Laboratory testing

   B) Comprehensive medical workup

   C) Duration and pervasiveness of worry

   D) Family history of anxiety

4. A newly diagnosed GAD patient asks about treatment options. Which initial approach has the strongest evidence base?

   A) Benzodiazepines alone

   B) Cognitive behavioral therapy and/or SSRI/SNRI

C) Alternative medicine only

D) Supportive therapy alone

5. A patient with GAD reports worsening symptoms despite SSRI treatment for 8 weeks at an adequate dose. What is the most appropriate next step?

A) Immediately switch to a different medication

B) Add a benzodiazepine

C) Evaluate adherence, optimize dose, consider augmentation

D) Discontinue medication entirely

8.2 Panic Disorder

6. A 25-year-old presents to the emergency room with sudden onset of racing heart, shortness of breath, sweating, and fear of dying. This is the third similar episode in two weeks, and the patient now fears having another attack. Medical workup is negative. Which diagnosis is most appropriate?

A) Acute Stress Disorder

B) Panic Disorder

C) Medical emergency

D) Generalized Anxiety Disorder

7. A patient reports panic symptoms only when giving presentations at work. Which diagnosis is most likely?

A) Panic Disorder

B) Social Anxiety Disorder with panic attacks

C) Specific Phobia

D) Generalized Anxiety Disorder with panic attacks

8. During evaluation of recurrent panic attacks, which clinical feature is MOST important in determining prognosis and treatment planning?

A) Age of onset

B) Presence and severity of agoraphobic avoidance

C) Family history

D) Number of symptoms during attacks

9. What is the most appropriate initial treatment approach for newly diagnosed Panic Disorder?

   A) Long-term benzodiazepine use

   B) CBT focused on panic and/or SSRI

   C) Beta blockers only

   D) Supportive counseling alone

10. A patient with Panic Disorder develops increasing avoidance of public places. Which intervention should be prioritized?

    A) Increase antidepressant dose only

    B) Early exposure therapy with continued medication

    C) Switch to different medication class

    D) Add long-term benzodiazepine

8.3 Specific Phobias

11. A 28-year-old has intense fear of flying that causes complete avoidance of air travel, impacting their career advancement. Despite recognizing the fear is excessive, they cannot overcome it. Which diagnosis is most appropriate?

    A) Panic Disorder with Agoraphobia

    B) Generalized Anxiety Disorder

    C) Specific Phobia, situational type

    D) Adjustment Disorder with anxiety

12. During assessment of a patient with fear of heights, which feature is MOST important for diagnosing a specific phobia?

    A) Family history of similar fears

    B) Degree of functional impairment

    C) Age of onset

D) Physical symptoms during exposure

13. A patient presents with severe fear of dogs after a recent dog bite. What is the most crucial factor in differentiating between normal fear and specific phobia?

A) Severity of the original trauma

B) Time since the incident

C) Degree of impairment and avoidance

D) Physical symptoms when seeing dogs

14. What is the most appropriate first-line treatment for specific phobia according to current evidence?

A) SSRI medication

B) Exposure-based therapy

C) Psychodynamic therapy

D) Benzodiazepines as needed

15. A patient with blood-injection phobia requires regular medical procedures. Which specific intervention should be prioritized?

A) Applied muscle tension technique

B) Systematic desensitization only

C) Anxiolytic medication alone

D) Cognitive restructuring only

8.4 Social Anxiety Disorder

16. A 22-year-old student avoids class presentations, speaking in groups, and eating in public due to intense fear of embarrassment. Academic performance is declining despite good understanding of material. Which diagnosis is most appropriate?

A) Specific Phobia

B) Panic Disorder

C) Social Anxiety Disorder

D) Avoidant Personality Disorder

17. A patient reports anxiety only when performing music in public, but not in other social situations. Which diagnostic specification is most appropriate?

A) Social Anxiety Disorder, generalized type

B) Social Anxiety Disorder, performance only

C) Specific Phobia

D) Panic Disorder with specific trigger

18. In evaluating treatment options for Social Anxiety Disorder, a patient expresses interest in both medication and therapy. What is the most appropriate initial approach?

A) Combined SSRI and CBT from the start

B) Either SSRI or CBT alone initially

C) Benzodiazepines as primary treatment

D) Beta blockers for all situations

19. A college student with Social Anxiety Disorder has started avoiding all classes. Which intervention should be prioritized?

A) Medical leave from school

B) Gradual exposure with skills training

C) Immediate benzodiazepine prescription

D) Change to online classes only

20. During assessment of a patient with possible Social Anxiety Disorder, which feature is MOST important to evaluate?

A) Childhood temperament

B) Impact on current functioning and quality of life

C) Family history

D) Intelligence level

8.5 Agoraphobia

21. A patient has developed intense fear and avoidance of using public transportation, being in crowded places, and leaving home alone. These fears developed after experiencing a panic attack on a bus 6 months ago. Which diagnosis is most appropriate?

    A) Panic Disorder with Agoraphobia

    B) Agoraphobia without history of Panic Disorder

    C) Specific Phobia

    D) Generalized Anxiety Disorder

22. While assessing a patient with agoraphobic symptoms, which clinical feature is MOST important for establishing prognosis?

    A) Number of avoided situations

    B) Presence of a support person

    C) Severity of panic symptoms

    D) Duration of symptoms

23. A homebound patient with severe Agoraphobia requires treatment. What is the most appropriate initial intervention?

    A) Start exposure therapy with outdoor sessions

    B) Begin treatment with home-based sessions and skills building

    C) Prescribe high-dose benzodiazepines

    D) Recommend inpatient treatment

24. In treating Agoraphobia, which therapeutic component should be prioritized early in treatment?

    A) Trauma processing

    B) Family therapy

    C) Safety behavior identification and reduction

    D) Cognitive restructuring only

25. A patient with Agoraphobia reports complete avoidance of all public places unless accompanied by their spouse. Which factor is MOST crucial to address in treatment?

    A) Spouse's anxiety level

    B) Dependency on safety person

    C) Patient's childhood history

    D) Current medication regimen

8.6 Separation Anxiety Disorder

26. A 7-year-old refuses to attend school, has frequent nightmares about losing parents, and becomes extremely distressed when parents leave. Symptoms have persisted for 5 months and significantly impact functioning. Which diagnosis is most appropriate?

    A) School Phobia

    B) Separation Anxiety Disorder

    C) Generalized Anxiety Disorder

    D) Adjustment Disorder

27. An adolescent with separation anxiety symptoms also shows depressive features. Which diagnostic approach is most appropriate?

    A) Focus only on most severe symptoms

    B) Evaluate criteria for both disorders independently

    C) Assume separation anxiety is secondary to depression

    D) Diagnose adjustment disorder only

28. During assessment of Separation Anxiety Disorder in a 6-year-old, which factor is MOST important to evaluate?

    A) Parental anxiety levels

    B) Impact on age-appropriate activities

    C) Intelligence level

    D) Sibling relationships

29. What is the most appropriate initial treatment approach for a young child with Separation Anxiety Disorder?

A) Individual play therapy only

B) Parent training and family-based CBT

C) Immediate medication

D) School-based counseling alone

30. A 12-year-old with Separation Anxiety Disorder refuses to sleep alone and frequently checks on parents during the night. Which intervention should be prioritized?

A) Sleep medication

B) Graduated exposure to independent sleeping

C) Family bed arrangement

D) Punishment for checking behaviors

Chapter 9: Obsessive-Compulsive and Related Disorders

9.1 Obsessive-Compulsive Disorder

1. A 25-year-old presents with intrusive thoughts about contamination leading to 3-hour daily cleaning rituals, significantly impacting work and relationships. The patient recognizes these concerns are excessive but cannot stop. Which diagnosis is most appropriate?

    A) Generalized Anxiety Disorder

    B) Obsessive-Compulsive Disorder

    C) Illness Anxiety Disorder

    D) Obsessive-Compulsive Personality Disorder

2. A patient with OCD reports both contamination fears and checking rituals. During initial treatment planning, which clinical feature is MOST important to assess?

    A) Family history of OCD

    B) Time spent on rituals and level of functional impairment

    C) Age of onset

    D) Presence of physical symptoms

3. During evaluation of OCD symptoms, a patient also reports depressive symptoms. Which sequence of treatment is most appropriate?

    A) Treat depression first, then OCD

    B) Address both conditions simultaneously

    C) Focus only on most severe condition

    D) Wait for spontaneous improvement

4. What is the most appropriate first-line treatment for moderate to severe OCD according to current evidence?

   A) Psychodynamic therapy

   B) SSRI medication and/or ERP (Exposure and Response Prevention)

   C) Supportive counseling

   D) Anxiolytics alone

5. A patient with OCD shows good insight about symptoms but has severe distress and compulsions. Which treatment approach should be prioritized?

   A) Cognitive therapy alone

   B) Exposure and Response Prevention (ERP)

   C) Social skills training

   D) Relaxation techniques only

9.2 Body Dysmorphic Disorder

6. A 19-year-old spends 4 hours daily checking perceived facial flaws in mirrors, has had multiple cosmetic procedures without satisfaction, and avoids social situations. Which diagnosis is most appropriate?

   A) Major Depressive Disorder

   B) Social Anxiety Disorder

   C) Body Dysmorphic Disorder

   D) Obsessive-Compulsive Disorder

7. During assessment of a patient with possible BDD who reports nose concerns, which clinical feature is MOST important to evaluate?

   A) Actual appearance of the nose

   B) Degree of preoccupation and functional impairment

   C) History of cosmetic procedures

   D) Family history of mental illness

8. A patient with BDD requests a referral for cosmetic surgery. What is the most appropriate response?

A) Provide immediate referral

B) Explain why psychiatric treatment should be prioritized

C) Agree to surgery if patient starts psychiatric medication

D) Ignore the request completely

9. What is the most appropriate first-line treatment approach for Body Dysmorphic Disorder?

A) SSRI medication and/or CBT with exposure

B) Supportive therapy alone

C) Cosmetic procedures

D) Anxiolytics as needed

10. A patient with BDD shows minimal insight into their condition. Which treatment consideration is MOST important?

A) Involuntary hospitalization

B) Focus on therapeutic alliance and gradual insight building

C) Immediate family intervention

D) Switch to intensive psychodynamic therapy

9.3 Hoarding Disorder

11. A 45-year-old lives alone in an apartment filled with newspapers, broken appliances, and random items collected over 20 years. Living spaces are unusable, and the patient can't discard items due to perceived value. Which diagnosis is most appropriate?

A) Obsessive-Compulsive Disorder

B) Hoarding Disorder

C) Collecting Hobby

D) Obsessive-Compulsive Personality Disorder

12. During assessment of hoarding behavior, which clinical feature is MOST important to evaluate?

    A) Total value of saved items

    B) Level of health and safety risk from clutter

    C) Family attitudes about hoarding

    D) Childhood collecting habits

13. A patient with Hoarding Disorder agrees to treatment but refuses home visits. What is the most appropriate initial intervention?

    A) Insist on home visit or refuse treatment

    B) Begin treatment in office while building trust

    C) Immediately involve family members

    D) Report to authorities

14. What is the most effective evidence-based treatment approach for Hoarding Disorder?

    A) Exposure therapy alone

    B) Specialized CBT for hoarding with home visits

    C) Regular cleaning service

    D) Medication only

15. A patient with severe hoarding creates fire hazards in their home. Which intervention should be prioritized?

    A) Forced clean-out only

    B) Risk assessment and safety planning with community resources

    C) Immediate hospitalization

    D) Increase medication dose only

9.4 Trichotillomania (Hair-Pulling Disorder)

16. A 23-year-old female presents with noticeable hair loss and admits to repeatedly pulling out her hair when stressed, despite attempts to stop. She reports increasing distress about her appearance. Which diagnosis is most appropriate?

    A) Obsessive-Compulsive Disorder

    B) Trichotillomania

    C) Alopecia Areata

    D) Body Dysmorphic Disorder

17. During evaluation of hair pulling behavior, which clinical feature is MOST important to assess?

    A) Specific locations of hair pulling

    B) Presence of tension before and relief after pulling

    C) Impact on social/occupational functioning

    D) Family history of hair pulling

18. A patient with Trichotillomania reports both focused and automatic pulling. What is the most appropriate initial treatment approach?

    A) SSRI medication alone

    B) Habit reversal training with stimulus control

    C) Supportive therapy only

    D) Antipsychotic medication

19. Which comorbid condition should be carefully assessed in a patient with Trichotillomania who reports ingesting pulled hair?

    A) Trichophagia and risk of trichobezoar

    B) Generalized anxiety only

    C) Depression only

    D) Social anxiety only

20. A teenager with Trichotillomania shows treatment resistance. Which factor is MOST important to re-evaluate?

A) Early childhood trauma

B) Current psychosocial stressors and maintaining factors

C) Genetic predisposition

D) Diet and exercise habits

9.5 Excoriation (Skin-Picking) Disorder

21. A 30-year-old presents with multiple skin lesions from chronic picking, causing significant distress and scarring. She can't stop despite numerous attempts and infections. Which diagnosis is most appropriate?

A) Self-Injurious Behavior

B) Excoriation (Skin-Picking) Disorder

C) Obsessive-Compulsive Disorder

D) Dermatitis Artefacta

22. During assessment of skin-picking behavior, which factor is MOST important to evaluate?

A) Family history of skin conditions

B) Medical complications and infection risk

C) Preferred picking tools

D) Childhood onset

23. A patient reports skin picking occurs primarily while watching TV or studying. Which initial intervention is most appropriate?

A) Immediate SSRI prescription

B) Habit reversal and stimulus control strategies

C) Intensive psychodynamic therapy

D) Cognitive restructuring only

24. What is the most appropriate way to address wound care in Excoriation Disorder treatment?

    A) Ignore wound care to avoid reinforcing behavior

    B) Include wound care while maintaining focus on picking reduction

    C) Focus exclusively on wound treatment

    D) Refer to dermatologist only

25. A patient with Excoriation Disorder shows minimal improvement with behavior therapy alone. Which treatment modification is most appropriate?

    A) Discontinue all treatment

    B) Consider combined approach with SSRI

    C) Switch to exclusive medication management

    D) Add exposure therapy only

Chapter 10: Trauma- and Stressor-Related Disorders

10.1 Post-Traumatic Stress Disorder (PTSD)

1. A 35-year-old veteran presents with nightmares, flashbacks, hypervigilance, and emotional numbing 6 months after combat exposure. He avoids anything military-related and has difficulty maintaining relationships. Which diagnosis is most appropriate?

   A) Acute Stress Disorder

   B) Post-Traumatic Stress Disorder

   C) Adjustment Disorder

   D) Generalized Anxiety Disorder

2. Which initial assessment focus is MOST crucial when evaluating a patient with suspected PTSD?

   A) Detailed trauma narrative

   B) Current safety and suicidal risk

   C) Family psychiatric history

   D) Childhood development history

3. A patient with PTSD reports both nightmares and insomnia. What is the most appropriate initial treatment approach?

   A) Immediate exposure therapy

   B) Trauma-focused CBT and consideration of medication

   C) Sleep medication alone

   D) Supportive counseling only

4. Which symptom pattern is MOST important to assess in differentiating PTSD from Acute Stress Disorder?

    A) Type of trauma exposure

    B) Severity of symptoms

    C) Duration of symptoms

    D) Age at trauma exposure

5. A PTSD patient reports increasing alcohol use to manage symptoms. Which intervention should be prioritized?

    A) Focus only on PTSD treatment

    B) Address both PTSD and substance use concurrently

    C) Treat substance use first, then PTSD

    D) Refer to separate providers for each condition

10.2 Acute Stress Disorder

6. A 28-year-old presents with severe anxiety, flashbacks, and dissociative symptoms two weeks after witnessing a fatal car accident. Sleep is disrupted and work performance is affected. Which diagnosis is most appropriate?

    A) Post-Traumatic Stress Disorder

    B) Acute Stress Disorder

    C) Adjustment Disorder

    D) Major Depressive Disorder

7. During assessment of Acute Stress Disorder, which timeframe is MOST important to establish for diagnosis?

    A) Symptoms present for at least 6 months

    B) Symptoms for 3 days to 1 month post-trauma

    C) Symptoms for more than 1 month

    D) Immediate onset post-trauma only

8. A patient presents with acute stress symptoms after a natural disaster. Which intervention should be prioritized in the first few days?

A) Immediate trauma processing

B) Practical support and safety planning

C) Exposure therapy

D) Antidepressant medication

9. Which factor is MOST predictive of progression from Acute Stress Disorder to PTSD?

A) Prior psychiatric history

B) Severity of initial symptoms and avoidance

C) Age at trauma exposure

D) Gender of the patient

10. A patient with Acute Stress Disorder shows significant dissociative symptoms. What is the most appropriate treatment approach?

A) Immediate trauma narrative work

B) Grounding techniques and symptom management

C) High-dose antipsychotics

D) Intensive exposure therapy

10.3 Adjustment Disorders

11. A 42-year-old develops anxiety, depressed mood, and insomnia following job loss 6 weeks ago. Symptoms exceed expected reaction but don't meet criteria for major depression. Which diagnosis is most appropriate?

A) Major Depressive Disorder

B) Adjustment Disorder with mixed anxiety and depressed mood

C) Generalized Anxiety Disorder

D) Acute Stress Disorder

12. During assessment of Adjustment Disorder, which clinical feature is MOST important to establish?

    A) Family history of mental illness

    B) Temporal relationship between stressor and symptoms

    C) Childhood trauma history

    D) Personality traits

13. A patient presents with adjustment disorder following divorce. Within what timeframe must symptoms begin after the stressor to meet diagnostic criteria?

    A) Within 1 week

    B) Within 3 months

    C) Within 6 months

    D) Within 1 year

14. What is the most appropriate initial treatment approach for Adjustment Disorder?

    A) Long-term psychodynamic therapy

    B) Brief supportive therapy and problem-solving

    C) Immediate medication

    D) Intensive CBT

15. Which factor is MOST important in differentiating Adjustment Disorder from a major depressive episode?

    A) Presence of sleep problems

    B) Severity and number of symptoms

    C) Duration of symptoms

    D) Type of stressor

10.4 Reactive Attachment Disorder

16. A 3-year-old child shows minimal social and emotional responsiveness, rarely seeks comfort when distressed, and has limited positive affect. History reveals severe neglect in early life. Which diagnosis is most appropriate?

    A) Autism Spectrum Disorder

    B) Reactive Attachment Disorder

    C) Social Anxiety Disorder

    D) Adjustment Disorder

17. During evaluation of possible Reactive Attachment Disorder, which environmental factor is MOST crucial to assess?

    A) Parental education level

    B) History of insufficient caregiving

    C) Socioeconomic status

    D) Genetic predisposition

18. What age criterion must be met for diagnosing Reactive Attachment Disorder?

    A) Symptoms before age 5 years

    B) Onset after age 5 years

    C) Diagnosis only in adolescence

    D) No age requirement

19. Which intervention should be prioritized in treating a child with Reactive Attachment Disorder?

    A) Individual play therapy only

    B) Ensuring stable, responsive caregiving environment

    C) Medication management

    D) Strict behavioral modification

20. A foster child with RAD shows improvement in a stable placement. Which factor is MOST important for continued progress?

    A) Regular IQ testing

    B) Support and education for current caregivers

C) Focus on past trauma

D) Peer group therapy

10.5 Disinhibited Social Engagement Disorder

21. A 4-year-old child with a history of institutional care readily approaches and shows physical affection with strangers, lacks normal social boundaries, and willingly leaves with unfamiliar adults. Which diagnosis is most appropriate?

    A) Attention-Deficit/Hyperactivity Disorder

    B) Disinhibited Social Engagement Disorder

    C) Autism Spectrum Disorder

    D) Oppositional Defiant Disorder

22. In differentiating DSED from normal sociability in young children, which feature is MOST important?

    A) Child's IQ level

    B) Lack of appropriate wariness of strangers

    C) General activity level

    D) Language development

23. Which historical factor is MOST essential to establish for diagnosing DSED?

    A) Family history of mental illness

    B) Pattern of inadequate early caregiving

    C) Birth complications

    D) Developmental milestones

24. What is the most appropriate initial treatment focus for DSED?

    A) Medication management

    B) Establishing consistent caregiving and safety training

    C) Peer group socialization

    D) Academic interventions

25. Which safety concern should be prioritized when working with a child with DSED?

A) Risk of elopement with strangers

B) Academic performance

C) Peer relationships

D) Sleep patterns

Chapter 11: **Somatic Symptom and Related Disorders**

11.1 Somatic Symptom Disorder

1. A 35-year-old presents with multiple physical complaints (fatigue, pain, GI symptoms) for over one year. Medical workup is negative, but the patient shows excessive anxiety about symptoms and spends significant time researching diseases. Which diagnosis is most appropriate?

   A) Illness Anxiety Disorder

   B) Somatic Symptom Disorder

   C) Major Depressive Disorder

   D) Generalized Anxiety Disorder

2. During assessment of Somatic Symptom Disorder, which feature is MOST important to evaluate?

   A) Number of physical symptoms

   B) Impact of health concerns on daily functioning

   C) Results of medical tests

   D) Family history of medical conditions

3. A patient with suspected Somatic Symptom Disorder requests another specialist referral. What is the most appropriate response?

   A) Refuse all medical workup

   B) Validate concerns while maintaining consistent treatment approach

   C) Immediately refer to all requested specialists

   D) Tell patient symptoms are "all in their head"

4. What is the most appropriate initial treatment approach for Somatic Symptom Disorder?

   A) Antidepressant medication only

   B) CBT focused on coping with symptoms

   C) Extensive medical testing

   D) Multiple specialty referrals

5. Which factor is MOST important in differentiating Somatic Symptom Disorder from a medical condition?

   A) Number of symptoms

   B) Disproportionate thoughts/behaviors about symptoms

   C) Absence of medical findings

   D) Duration of symptoms

11.2 Illness Anxiety Disorder

6. A 28-year-old is preoccupied with the possibility of having cancer despite no physical symptoms and normal medical evaluations. They check their body multiple times daily and frequently research diseases online. Which diagnosis is most appropriate?

   A) Somatic Symptom Disorder

   B) Illness Anxiety Disorder

   C) Obsessive-Compulsive Disorder

   D) Generalized Anxiety Disorder

7. Which feature is MOST important in differentiating Illness Anxiety Disorder from Somatic Symptom Disorder?

   A) Level of anxiety

   B) Absence of significant physical symptoms

   C) Duration of concerns

   D) Number of doctor visits

8. A patient with Illness Anxiety Disorder seeks frequent medical reassurance. Which therapeutic approach is most appropriate?

A) Provide repeated medical testing

B) Cognitive restructuring and response prevention

C) Ignore health concerns completely

D) Daily physical examinations

9. During assessment of Illness Anxiety Disorder, which clinical feature should be prioritized?

A) Childhood medical history

B) Risk of self-harm and safety concerns

C) Family medical history

D) Educational level

10. What is the most appropriate way to address internet health research with an Illness Anxiety patient?

A) Ban all medical research

B) Set limits while teaching critical evaluation skills

C) Encourage unlimited research

D) Ignore the behavior

11.3 Conversion Disorder (Functional Neurological Symptom Disorder)

11. A 32-year-old develops sudden leg weakness and tremors after a stressful event. Neurological examination and testing are inconsistent with known medical conditions. Which diagnosis is most appropriate?

A) Multiple Sclerosis

B) Conversion Disorder

C) Malingering

D) Somatic Symptom Disorder

12. During assessment of possible Conversion Disorder, which clinical feature is MOST important to evaluate?

   A) Childhood trauma history

   B) Inconsistency with recognized neurological disease

   C) Presence of depression

   D) Family history of neurological conditions

13. A patient presents with conversion symptoms affecting gait. What is the most appropriate initial treatment approach?

   A) Immediately confront about psychological causes

   B) Physical therapy while addressing psychosocial factors

   C) Psychiatric medication only

   D) Tell patient symptoms are not real

14. Which factor is MOST important in determining prognosis in Conversion Disorder?

   A) Age of onset

   B) Duration of symptoms before treatment

   C) Type of symptoms

   D) Gender of patient

15. A patient with Conversion Disorder shows symptom escalation during examination. Which clinical approach is most appropriate?

   A) Discharge immediately

   B) Matter-of-fact, non-judgmental examination

   C) Increase medication doses

   D) Order repeated diagnostic tests

11.4 Factitious Disorder

16. A patient repeatedly presents with different acute medical complaints, provides inconsistent medical histories, and becomes hostile when records are requested. Previous hospitalizations reveal pattern of self-induced symptoms. Which diagnosis is most appropriate?

    A) Somatic Symptom Disorder

    B) Factitious Disorder

    C) Malingering

    D) Conversion Disorder

17. In evaluating suspected Factitious Disorder, which clinical feature is MOST important to assess?

    A) Family psychiatric history

    B) Pattern of deceptive behavior and intentional symptom production

    C) Childhood medical history

    D) Current life stressors

18. When Factitious Disorder is suspected, what is the most appropriate initial management approach?

    A) Immediate confrontation about deception

    B) Maintain therapeutic alliance while setting clear boundaries

    C) Refuse all medical care

    D) Notify all regional hospitals

19. Which factor is MOST important in differentiating Factitious Disorder from Malingering?

    A) Severity of symptoms

    B) Conscious motivation for external rewards

    C) Type of symptoms presented

    D) Age of onset

20. A patient with confirmed Factitious Disorder requires medical treatment for genuine illness. Which approach is most appropriate?

A) Deny all treatment

B) Provide coordinated care with clear boundaries

C) Refer to another facility

D) Treat only with maximum security measures

Chapter 12: **Other Categories of Disorders**

12.1 Sleep-Wake Disorders

1. A 40-year-old reports chronic difficulty falling asleep and maintaining sleep for 6 months, causing significant daytime fatigue and work impairment. No medical conditions or substances explain symptoms. Which diagnosis is most appropriate?

    A) Primary Insomnia Disorder

    B) Adjustment Sleep Disorder

    C) Sleep Apnea

    D) Circadian Rhythm Sleep Disorder

2. During evaluation of chronic insomnia, which assessment tool is MOST important to implement?

    A) Immediate sleep study

    B) Two-week sleep diary

    C) Family history only

    D) Personality testing

3. A patient presents with sudden episodes of muscle weakness triggered by strong emotions. Which sleep disorder should be suspected?

    A) Narcolepsy Type 1

    B) Sleep Apnea

    C) Insomnia Disorder

    D) REM Sleep Behavior Disorder

4. What is the most appropriate first-line treatment for chronic insomnia according to current guidelines?

   A) Long-term benzodiazepine use

   B) Cognitive Behavioral Therapy for Insomnia (CBT-I)

   C) Over-the-counter sleep aids

   D) Melatonin only

5. A patient with insomnia shows evidence of depression. Which treatment approach is most appropriate?

   A) Treat insomnia only

   B) Address both conditions concurrently

   C) Focus only on depression

   D) Refer to separate specialists

12.2 Personality Disorders

6. A 25-year-old shows a persistent pattern of unstable relationships, intense fear of abandonment, recurrent suicidal behavior, and unstable identity. Symptoms began in adolescence. Which diagnosis is most appropriate?

   A) Major Depressive Disorder

   B) Borderline Personality Disorder

   C) Bipolar Disorder

   D) Histrionic Personality Disorder

7. During assessment of a possible personality disorder, which clinical feature is MOST important to establish?

   A) Current symptoms only

   B) Long-standing pattern of behavior since adolescence/early adulthood

   C) Recent life stressors

   D) Family psychiatric history

8. A patient with Borderline Personality Disorder presents with suicidal thoughts. What is the most appropriate initial intervention?

   A) Immediate hospitalization

   B) Risk assessment and development of safety plan

   C) Start medications only

   D) Refer to another provider

9. What is the most appropriate evidence-based treatment approach for Borderline Personality Disorder?

   A) Medication management only

   B) Dialectical Behavior Therapy (DBT) or other specialized psychotherapy

   C) Supportive counseling alone

   D) Crisis intervention only

10. In treating a patient with Narcissistic Personality Disorder, which therapeutic factor is MOST important?

    A) Continuous confrontation

    B) Maintaining empathic stance while setting boundaries

    C) Immediate interpretation of defenses

    D) Focus on childhood only

12.3 Neurocognitive Disorders

11. A 72-year-old shows progressive memory decline, word-finding difficulties, and impaired daily functioning over the past year. No sudden onset or stroke history. Which diagnosis is most appropriate?

    A) Age-related memory decline

    B) Major Neurocognitive Disorder due to possible Alzheimer's

    C) Mild Cognitive Impairment

    D) Delirium

12. During evaluation of cognitive decline, which assessment approach is MOST important initially?

    A) Immediate brain MRI

    B) Cognitive screening plus functional assessment

    C) Genetic testing

    D) Psychiatric history only

13. A patient develops sudden confusion, fluctuating attention, and disorientation in the hospital. Which diagnosis should be prioritized?

    A) Dementia

    B) Delirium

    C) Depression

    D) Anxiety Disorder

14. What is the most appropriate first step in treating newly diagnosed Major Neurocognitive Disorder?

    A) Immediate antipsychotic medication

    B) Safety assessment and support system evaluation

    C) Memory medication only

    D) Nursing home placement

15. Which factor is MOST important in differentiating Major from Mild Neurocognitive Disorder?

    A) Age of onset

    B) Impact on independent functioning

    C) Presence of memory complaints

    D) Family history

12.4 Feeding and Eating Disorders

16. A 19-year-old female presents with BMI of 16.5, intense fear of gaining weight, body image distortion, and amenorrhea. Which diagnosis is most appropriate?

    A) Bulimia Nervosa

    B) Anorexia Nervosa

    C) Avoidant/Restrictive Food Intake Disorder

    D) Binge Eating Disorder

17. During assessment of an eating disorder, which medical complication should be prioritized for evaluation?

    A) Skin changes

    B) Cardiac complications

    C) Dental erosion

    D) Hair loss

18. A patient with Anorexia Nervosa resists weight gain despite medical complications. What is the most appropriate next step?

    A) Respect patient's autonomy

    B) Evaluate for higher level of care

    C) Increase therapy sessions only

    D) Start medications only

19. Which treatment approach has the strongest evidence base for Bulimia Nervosa?

    A) Cognitive Behavioral Therapy

    B) Supportive counseling

    C) Medication alone

    D) Family therapy for adults

20. A patient with an eating disorder shows signs of suicide risk. Which intervention should take precedence?

    A) Focus only on eating disorder

    B) Immediate safety assessment and intervention

C) Increase medication dose

D) Refer to another provider

12.5 Sexual Dysfunctions

21. A 45-year-old male reports persistent difficulty maintaining erections for 6 months, causing significant distress. Medical evaluation shows mild hypertension. Which diagnosis is most appropriate?

    A) Erectile Disorder

    B) Male Hypoactive Sexual Desire Disorder

    C) Performance Anxiety

    D) Adjustment Disorder

22. During evaluation of sexual dysfunction, which aspect is MOST important to assess initially?

    A) Relationship satisfaction only

    B) Medical conditions and medications

    C) Childhood experiences

    D) Cultural factors only

23. A patient reports loss of sexual desire affecting relationship but no distress about it. Which diagnostic consideration is most appropriate?

    A) Sexual Desire Disorder

    B) Consider normal variation

    C) Major Depression

    D) Anxiety Disorder

24. What is the most appropriate initial approach for treating Female Sexual Interest/Arousal Disorder?

    A) Immediate medication

    B) Comprehensive biopsychosocial approach

    C) Relationship therapy only

    D) Hormonal treatment only

25. A couple presents with sexual difficulties. Which treatment approach is most appropriate?

    A) Individual therapy only

    B) Combined individual and couple therapy as needed

    C) Medication management only

    D) Focus exclusively on one partner

12.6 Gender Dysphoria

26. An adolescent reports persistent distress about gender assigned at birth, strong desire to be treated as another gender, and significant impairment in functioning. Duration is 2 years. Which diagnosis is most appropriate?

    A) Gender Dysphoria

    B) Adjustment Disorder

    C) Body Dysmorphic Disorder

    D) Identity Problem

27. During evaluation of Gender Dysphoria, which clinical feature is MOST important to assess?

    A) Sexual orientation

    B) Level of distress and functional impairment

    C) Family history

    D) Early childhood experiences only

28. What is the most appropriate initial treatment approach for an adolescent with Gender Dysphoria?

    A) Immediate medical intervention

    B) Comprehensive evaluation and support

    C) Wait until adulthood

    D) Family therapy only

29. During treatment planning for Gender Dysphoria, which factor should be prioritized?

    A) Personal goals and timeline for transition

    B) Family's wishes only

    C) Immediate medical transition

    D) Societal expectations

30. Which approach is most appropriate when working with a young person exploring gender identity?

    A) Rush to diagnosis

    B) Affirming support while allowing exploration

    C) Discourage exploration

    D) Immediate referral for medical intervention

12.7 Disruptive, Impulse-Control, and Conduct Disorders

31. A 13-year-old shows persistent pattern of aggression toward others, destruction of property, frequent lying, and stealing over the past year. No prior history of behavioral problems. Which diagnosis is most appropriate?

    A) Oppositional Defiant Disorder

    B) Conduct Disorder

    C) ADHD

    D) Adjustment Disorder

32. When evaluating aggressive behavior in an adolescent, which factor is MOST important to assess?

    A) Academic performance only

    B) Risk of harm to self or others

    C) Family income level

D) Peer relationships only

33. A 15-year-old shows severe conduct problems and lack of empathy/remorse. Which specifier should be considered?

A) Limited prosocial emotions

B) High functioning

C) Socially adjusted

D) Academic success

34. What is the most appropriate evidence-based treatment approach for Conduct Disorder?

A) Medication only

B) Parent management training and multimodal intervention

C) Individual therapy only

D) School intervention only

35. During treatment of a teen with severe conduct problems, which intervention should be prioritized?

A) Focus only on past trauma

B) Safety planning and risk management

C) Academic support only

D) Peer group therapy only

12.8 Substance-Related and Addictive Disorders

36. A 28-year-old shows increased alcohol tolerance, withdrawal symptoms, unsuccessful attempts to cut down, and continued use despite job problems. Which diagnosis is most appropriate?

A) Alcohol Use Disorder, Moderate-Severe

B) Alcohol Use Disorder, Mild

C) Alcohol Abuse

D) Problem Drinking

37. During assessment of substance use, which aspect should be prioritized first?

    A) Family history of addiction

    B) Immediate medical risks and withdrawal potential

    C) Employment status

    D) Legal history

38. A patient reports daily opioid use and wants to stop. What is the most appropriate initial intervention?

    A) Immediate cessation of use

    B) Medically supervised withdrawal planning

    C) Outpatient counseling only

    D) Refer to NA meetings only

39. Which factor is MOST important in determining level of care for substance treatment?

    A) Patient preference only

    B) Severity, risk, and recovery environment

    C) Insurance coverage

    D) Distance to treatment facility

40. A patient with alcohol use disorder reports depression. Which treatment approach is most appropriate?

    A) Treat alcohol use only

    B) Address both conditions concurrently

    C) Focus on depression first

    D) Wait for sustained sobriety

Answers to Interactive Questions

Thank you for completing this comprehensive section of practice questions. This interactive learning experience has covered key diagnostic criteria, clinical presentations, and treatment approaches across major psychiatric disorders based on DSM-5-TR guidelines.

Simply scan the QR code below to access our digital platform. Upon login, you will receive:

1. A downloadable PDF of all your previous responses

2. Regular updates with new clinical scenarios and evidence-based guidelines

Enhance your learning experience by combining traditional study methods with our digital resources, designed to support your preparation for clinical practice and board examinations.

Note: Access to the digital platform is included with your purchase of this text.

Section 3:
Real-World Clinical Cases

Introduction to Section 3: The Value of Case Studies in Clinical Practice

Case studies serve as powerful tools in clinical practice, bridging the gap between theoretical knowledge and real-world application. They allow clinicians, students, and mental health professionals to engage with complex diagnostic and therapeutic scenarios in a controlled, reflective way. By examining diverse cases, clinicians develop a deeper understanding of the nuances within each disorder, refine their diagnostic skills, and practice the decision-making processes essential to effective patient care.

The value of case studies lies in their ability to:
- **Enhance Diagnostic Skills**: Each case offers insight into applying DSM-5-TR criteria to real patients. By reviewing symptoms, patient history, and context, clinicians learn to identify key diagnostic features and distinguish between similar disorders.

- **Illustrate Differential Diagnosis**: Case studies help clinicians understand how to systematically rule out other potential diagnoses, consider comorbidities, and appreciate the complexity of overlapping symptoms. This approach reduces misdiagnoses and sharpens the ability to handle ambiguous cases.

- **Support Evidence-Based Treatment Planning**: Through detailed case outcomes, professionals gain exposure to treatment modalities and interventions. They see how different therapeutic strategies are applied and learn to adapt these strategies to patients' individual needs.

- **Promote Clinical Reflection and Empathy**: By exploring the patient's perspective, case studies encourage clinicians to consider the lived experience of mental health disorders. This holistic view supports a compassionate, patient-centered approach that values both clinical efficacy and the human aspect of care.

This section provides a series of carefully structured case studies across major diagnostic categories. Each case is designed to offer hands-on practice in diagnosis and to foster a deeper understanding of the challenges and solutions encountered in mental health care. Whether you are a student or a seasoned clinician, these cases are intended to enhance your clinical judgment, sharpen your skills, and provide a meaningful framework for effective patient care.

Chapter 13: **Clinical Cases in Neurodevelopmental Disorders**

Introduction to Neurodevelopmental Disorders

Neurodevelopmental disorders are a group of conditions characterized by developmental deficits that produce impairments in personal, social, academic, or occupational functioning. Emerging in early childhood and typically identified before school age, these disorders can impact multiple areas, including cognition, behavior, and communication. Their presentation varies widely in severity, with some individuals experiencing mild impairments and others facing significant challenges that affect daily functioning and quality of life.

The DSM-5-TR outlines several primary neurodevelopmental disorders, each with distinct diagnostic criteria but often overlapping features. Disorders such as Autism Spectrum Disorder (ASD) and Attention-Deficit/Hyperactivity Disorder (ADHD), for instance, may present with both cognitive and behavioral symptoms, while others, like Communication Disorders or Intellectual Disability, primarily impact specific developmental domains. Understanding the unique presentation of each disorder, along with the nuanced differences between them, is crucial for accurate diagnosis and effective treatment planning.

In clinical practice, diagnosing neurodevelopmental disorders involves not only assessing symptoms but also considering the child's developmental history, family context, and educational environment. Early and accurate diagnosis is essential, as timely intervention can substantially improve long-term outcomes. Clinicians rely on a combination of behavioral assessments, standardized tests, and input from caregivers and educators to create a comprehensive diagnostic profile.

This chapter presents a series of real-world clinical cases across the neurodevelopmental disorder spectrum, offering insight into the diagnostic and therapeutic processes specific to each condition. Through these cases, clinicians and students will explore the complexities of assessing and managing neurodevelopmental disorders, developing the skills necessary to support individuals and their families effectively.

Case 13.1: Autism Spectrum Disorder

Patient Presentation
Patient: Matthew, a 7-year-old boy

Family Background: Matthew lives with his parents and younger sister in a suburban neighborhood. His parents, who both work full-time, are actively engaged in his care and are concerned about his limited social skills and communication difficulties. His mother reports that Matthew tends to avoid eye contact, shows minimal interest in playing with others, and becomes upset when his daily routines are altered.

Key Symptoms:
- **Social Interaction**: Matthew has a marked difficulty in social engagement. He avoids eye contact, shows limited facial expressions, and tends not to respond to others' attempts to interact, including family members.

- **Communication**: Matthew uses very few words, primarily echoing short phrases without engaging in meaningful conversation. He rarely initiates communication and uses language infrequently, often relying on pointing or leading his parents to an object he wants.

- **Behavioral Patterns**: Exhibits repetitive behaviors, such as hand-flapping when excited or stressed, and an intense preference for specific routines. Matthew becomes visibly distressed if his routines are disrupted or if he cannot carry his preferred object — a small blue toy car.

- **Cognitive and Motor Development**: Shows delays in cognitive skills, particularly in abstract reasoning and problem-solving tasks. Motor skills are largely age-appropriate, though he prefers activities that involve arranging or sorting objects rather than interactive play.

Symptom Evolution:

Matthew's parents began noticing developmental differences when he was around 2 years old. While other children at his daycare played together, he engaged in solitary play and displayed minimal interest in other children. Over time, his preference for routines and his limited communication have intensified, prompting his parents to seek a formal evaluation.

Previous Interventions or Diagnoses:

Matthew has no formal prior diagnosis. His pediatrician expressed mild concerns about his delayed social engagement and language skills at a routine check-up, recommending an evaluation to assess potential developmental concerns.

Clinical Decision-Making Process

DSM-5-TR Diagnostic Criteria Considered:
- **Persistent Deficits in Social Communication and Social Interaction**: Matthew demonstrates several core ASD features, including deficits in social-emotional reciprocity (e.g., limited responsiveness to social interactions), nonverbal communication difficulties (e.g., lack of eye contact and expressive gestures), and challenges in forming peer relationships.

- **Restricted and Repetitive Patterns of Behavior**: Repetitive behaviors, such as hand-flapping, and rigid adherence to specific routines were evident. His distress when routines are altered and his attachment to specific objects further support these criteria.

Exclusion of Other Diagnoses:
- **Social (Pragmatic) Communication Disorder**: This disorder was ruled out due to the presence of restricted interests and repetitive behaviors, which are characteristic of ASD but not of Social Communication Disorder.

- **Intellectual Disability**: Although Matthew displays mild cognitive delays, his specific social and behavioral patterns align more closely with Autism Spectrum Disorder. Intellectual Disability alone would not account for the restricted interests and social deficits observed.

Assessment Tools:
- **Autism Diagnostic Observation Schedule, Second Edition (ADOS-2)**: This standardized observation tool was administered to assess Matthew's social, communicative, and behavioral tendencies. Observations confirmed limited reciprocal social communication, restricted interests, and repetitive behaviors.

- **Child Behavior Checklist (CBCL)**: Administered to Matthew's parents to gather comprehensive information on his social behaviors, attention span, and emotional regulation. Results indicated significant concerns in social and communicative domains, consistent with ASD.

Family Involvement: The clinician worked closely with Matthew's parents to understand the impact of his symptoms on family dynamics and daily life. Through interviews, the clinician gathered details about his routines, preferences, and reactions in various social settings, which reinforced the diagnosis. The clinician also provided the family with an overview of the diagnostic process and the core symptoms of ASD, allowing them to understand the criteria and the rationale for the diagnosis.

Suggested Topics
- Application of ADOS-2 in Autism Spectrum Disorder diagnosis.
- Differentiating Autism Spectrum Disorder from Social (Pragmatic) Communication Disorder.
- Behavioral management strategies for children with ASD.
- Principles of Applied Behavior Analysis (ABA) therapy for social and communication skills improvement.

Case 13.2: Attention-Deficit/Hyperactivity Disorder (ADHD)

Patient Presentation
Patient: Joshua, an 8-year-old boy

Family Background: Joshua lives with his parents and two younger siblings in an urban neighborhood. Both parents work full-time, and he attends an after-school program until early evening. His teachers and parents report concerns over his academic performance and behavioral issues. At home, his parents note that Joshua has difficulty following instructions, often fails to complete chores, and frequently interrupts conversations.

Key Symptoms:
- **Inattention**: Joshua struggles to pay attention in class and is easily distracted by external stimuli. He often makes careless mistakes in his homework and school assignments, appearing to overlook details. His teachers observe that he rarely completes tasks on time and frequently loses items needed for school.

- **Hyperactivity and Impulsivity**: He displays signs of restlessness, such as fidgeting with his hands, tapping his feet, and frequently leaving his seat in the classroom. Joshua has difficulty waiting his turn and tends to interrupt others during activities and conversations, leading to conflicts with peers.

- **Social Interactions**: His impulsivity has affected his ability to make and maintain friendships. Other children sometimes avoid him because he often intrudes on their activities or becomes overly excited and boisterous during play.

Symptom Evolution:

Joshua's symptoms became noticeable when he started kindergarten. Teachers observed that he was frequently "on the go" and had trouble staying focused during lessons. By the second grade, his inability to sit still and follow classroom routines was affecting his academic performance. His parents attempted to support him with structured routines at home, but he continued to struggle with completing tasks and often became frustrated.

Previous Interventions or Diagnoses:

Joshua has no prior diagnosis, but his school recommended an evaluation due to his behavior. His parents previously consulted with the school counselor, who suggested behavioral strategies, yet these did not significantly improve his symptoms.

Clinical Decision-Making Process

DSM-5-TR Diagnostic Criteria Considered:
- **Inattention Symptoms**: Joshua meets multiple criteria within the inattention domain, including frequent careless mistakes, difficulty sustaining attention, failing to complete tasks, and losing essential items. These behaviors occur in multiple settings (home and school) and have been consistent for over six months.

- **Hyperactivity and Impulsivity Symptoms**: Joshua also displays symptoms of hyperactivity and impulsivity, such as leaving his seat, excessive fidgeting, and interrupting others. These behaviors are developmentally inappropriate and have caused notable interference in social and academic settings.

Exclusion of Other Diagnoses:
- **Oppositional Defiant Disorder (ODD)**: Although Joshua sometimes struggles with authority and becomes frustrated, his behavior is primarily marked by inattention and hyperactivity rather than defiance or argumentative tendencies, ruling out ODD.

- **Anxiety Disorders**: His symptoms do not align with anxiety disorders, as he does not exhibit pervasive worry or fear. His restlessness and impulsivity are not situation-specific but rather pervasive across various activities.

- **Specific Learning Disorder**: While Joshua's inattention impacts his academic performance, his cognitive abilities are age-appropriate, indicating that his difficulties stem from ADHD rather than a specific learning disorder.

Assessment Tools:
- **Conners 3 ADHD Rating Scale**: Completed by both his parents and teachers, this tool provided a detailed assessment of his attention, hyperactivity, and impulsivity. The results indicated significant concerns in areas consistent with ADHD.
- **Behavior Assessment System for Children (BASC-3)**: This instrument helped to assess Joshua's behavior from multiple perspectives, reinforcing concerns related to attention, impulse control, and difficulties in social interactions. These findings further supported the ADHD diagnosis.
- **Clinical Interview**: The clinician conducted a structured interview with Joshua's parents to gather comprehensive information on his developmental history, behavioral patterns, and the impact of symptoms on family dynamics. This interview highlighted the consistency of his symptoms across home and school environments, affirming the likelihood of ADHD.

Family Discussion: Joshua's parents were actively involved in the diagnostic process. The clinician explained the ADHD criteria in detail, discussing how his symptoms matched these criteria and explaining why other potential diagnoses were ruled out. His parents were also informed of the potential benefits of behavioral therapy and the role of family support in managing ADHD symptoms effectively. This discussion helped the family understand ADHD as a neurodevelopmental condition rather than simply "bad behavior," which facilitated a more supportive approach at home.

Suggested Topics
- Behavioral strategies and interventions for managing ADHD symptoms in children.
- Overview of ADHD rating scales and assessment tools, such as the Conners 3 and BASC-3.
- Differential diagnosis: distinguishing ADHD from other behavioral and learning disorders.

Case 13.3: Intellectual Disability

Patient Presentation
Patient: Emily, a 10-year-old girl

Family Background: Emily lives with her parents and older brother in a small, supportive community. Her mother stays at home, while her father works in construction. Emily attends a public school and has an Individualized Education Program (IEP) due to her learning and adaptive functioning challenges. Her parents report concerns about her academic performance, difficulty with social interactions, and limitations in daily life skills compared to her peers.

Key Symptoms:
- **Cognitive and Learning Delays**: Emily struggles with basic reading, writing, and math skills and performs below grade level across all academic subjects. She requires constant support to complete schoolwork and has difficulty following multi-step instructions.

- **Adaptive Functioning**: She shows limitations in everyday tasks. For example, Emily needs help with personal hygiene, managing her belongings, and understanding safety rules in unfamiliar situations. Her parents note she is easily confused by minor changes in routine, which increases her anxiety and stress.

- **Social and Communication Skills**: Emily tends to communicate in short phrases, and while her vocabulary is age-appropriate, she has difficulty understanding abstract concepts and social cues. She sometimes struggles to express her emotions appropriately and has few friends, primarily due to her limited understanding of social rules and norms.

Symptom Evolution:

Emily's developmental delays became noticeable during preschool when she struggled to reach cognitive and social milestones typical for her age. Teachers observed that she required repeated instructions and additional guidance to complete tasks. By age 6, her difficulties in both learning and adaptive skills became more apparent. Although she made progress with support services, her cognitive and adaptive limitations have remained significant and persistent.

Previous Interventions or Diagnoses:

Emily has had educational support since kindergarten and has been assessed by school psychologists, who initially noted her need for an IEP. No formal medical diagnosis had been given previously, though her family pursued further evaluation after her school recommended a comprehensive cognitive assessment to better understand her challenges.

Clinical Decision-Making Process

DSM-5-TR Diagnostic Criteria Considered:
- **Deficits in Intellectual Functioning**: Emily's performance in areas such as reasoning, problem-solving, and learning falls significantly below average for her age. This is documented through standardized testing, which shows a marked limitation in intellectual functioning.

- **Deficits in Adaptive Functioning**: Emily shows significant limitations in adaptive behavior across multiple areas. In daily living skills, she requires support for personal care and understanding basic safety, while her social limitations affect her ability to form age-appropriate friendships. These deficits impact her ability to function independently.

- **Onset During Developmental Period**: Emily's difficulties in intellectual and adaptive functioning have been evident since early childhood, meeting the DSM-5-TR criteria that these limitations must appear during the developmental period.

Exclusion of Other Diagnoses:
- **Learning Disorders**: While Emily demonstrates specific academic challenges, her broader limitations in intellectual and adaptive functioning indicate that her condition extends beyond a specific learning disorder.

- **Autism Spectrum Disorder (ASD)**: Although Emily shows some social and communication difficulties, she does not display repetitive behaviors or restricted interests characteristic of ASD. Her limitations are more consistent with Intellectual Disability rather than ASD.

Assessment Tools:
- **Wechsler Intelligence Scale for Children (WISC-V)**: This standardized IQ test was administered to assess Emily's cognitive abilities. Her scores indicated significantly below-average intellectual functioning across all major domains, supporting the diagnosis of Intellectual Disability.

- **Vineland Adaptive Behavior Scales (Vineland-3)**: Used to evaluate Emily's adaptive functioning in areas such as communication, daily living, and socialization. The results confirmed significant impairments in these areas, consistent with Intellectual Disability.

- **Behavior Rating Inventory of Executive Function (BRIEF)**: Completed by both parents and teachers, this tool provided further insight into Emily's executive functioning and adaptive behavior in school and home settings. The findings reinforced her need for high levels of support and supervision.

Family Discussion: Emily's parents were included throughout the evaluation process. The clinician discussed the DSM-5-TR criteria for Intellectual Disability, explaining Emily's intellectual and adaptive limitations in relation to her age group. The clinician emphasized the importance of ongoing support in both educational and daily living settings. Her parents expressed relief at having a clear diagnosis, which allowed them to better understand her needs and find appropriate resources for her continued development. They were given guidance on accessing community resources and support programs designed for children with Intellectual Disability.

Suggested Topics
- Understanding the role of adaptive functioning in Intellectual Disability.
- Overview of assessment tools for intellectual and adaptive functioning, including WISC-V and Vineland-3.
- Differentiating Intellectual Disability from specific learning disorders and developmental delays.

Case 13.4: Communication Disorder

Patient Presentation
Patient: Sarah, a 6-year-old girl

Family Background: Sarah lives with her mother, father, and an older brother in a suburban community. Her mother is a stay-at-home parent, while her father works full-time. Sarah's parents have noticed her struggle with language development compared to other children her age, impacting her confidence and social interactions, particularly in school. Her family describes her as a bright and curious child but one who has difficulty expressing herself verbally and understanding conversations fully.

Key Symptoms:

- **Delayed Language Development**: Sarah has difficulty with both expressive and receptive language. She often struggles to form full sentences and tends to use short, simple phrases to communicate. She also has trouble following complex instructions and understanding questions, particularly in a group setting.

- **Social and Emotional Impact**: Sarah becomes frustrated when she cannot communicate effectively, leading to frequent emotional outbursts. She appears withdrawn in social settings, often choosing solitary play over interacting with peers, as her limited language skills make it challenging to initiate and maintain conversations.

- **Pronunciation and Sentence Structure**: Sarah often mispronounces words and has difficulty with sentence structure, sometimes omitting words or using incorrect grammar. These issues are most apparent when she tries to describe events or share stories.

Symptom Evolution:

Sarah's parents first noticed delays in her language skills around age 3 when she was unable to speak in sentences like other children her age. Despite receiving support from her family and her preschool teachers, her language development continued to lag behind that of her peers. By kindergarten, her challenges became more pronounced, particularly as social and academic demands increased. This prompted her school to recommend a formal language evaluation.

Previous Interventions or Diagnoses:

Sarah has received speech therapy intermittently since the age of 4, focusing on basic language skills and pronunciation. While this therapy has helped her make some progress, her parents report that her language skills remain significantly delayed. She has not previously been diagnosed with a specific communication disorder.

Clinical Decision-Making Process

DSM-5-TR Diagnostic Criteria Considered:
- **Language Disorder Criteria**: Sarah meets several DSM-5-TR criteria for Language Disorder, a specific type of Communication Disorder. These include persistent difficulties with language acquisition and use, limited vocabulary, and difficulties with sentence structure and grammar. These challenges are not attributable to sensory impairments, motor dysfunction, or intellectual disability, and have significantly impacted her daily communication.

- **Impact on Functioning**: Sarah's communication difficulties affect her social interactions, academic performance, and emotional well-being, meeting the criteria that the disorder must interfere with functional communication.

Exclusion of Other Diagnoses:
- **Speech Sound Disorder**: While Sarah has some issues with pronunciation, her difficulties are primarily related to language comprehension and sentence structure, which are characteristic of Language Disorder rather than Speech Sound Disorder.

- **Autism Spectrum Disorder (ASD)**: Although Sarah has challenges with communication, she does not display restricted interests, repetitive behaviors, or significant social engagement difficulties beyond her language issues, which allows for ruling out ASD.

- **Intellectual Disability**: Sarah's cognitive abilities in non-language areas are age-appropriate, indicating that her language difficulties are not secondary to an overall intellectual impairment.

Assessment Tools:
- **Clinical Evaluation of Language Fundamentals (CELF-5)**: This assessment was used to evaluate Sarah's receptive and expressive language skills. Results indicated significant delays in both areas, reinforcing the likelihood of a Language Disorder.

- **Peabody Picture Vocabulary Test (PPVT)**: The PPVT provided insight into Sarah's vocabulary development, revealing a limited range of vocabulary words for her age group.

- **Expressive Vocabulary Test (EVT-2)**: Administered to assess her ability to use words in meaningful ways, the EVT-2 results supported the diagnosis, highlighting specific gaps in Sarah's vocabulary and sentence formulation skills.

Family Discussion: The clinician met with Sarah's parents to discuss the Language Disorder diagnosis and explain how it differs from typical language delays. The clinician emphasized the importance of continuing speech therapy with a focus on vocabulary building, sentence structure, and conversational skills. Sarah's parents were provided with information on additional language interventions and activities they could incorporate at home to support her language development.

Suggested Topics

- Overview of Language Disorder and differentiating it from other Communication Disorders.
- Role of speech and language therapy in treating Language Disorder.
- Key assessment tools for evaluating language development, including CELF-5 and PPVT.

Case 13.5: Specific Learning Disorder

Patient Presentation

Patient: Liam, a 9-year-old boy

Family Background: Liam lives with his parents and younger sister in an urban area. Both parents are professionals, and they are very involved in Liam's academic life. Since starting school, Liam has struggled academically, particularly in reading and mathematics, and his teachers have observed that he becomes easily frustrated with schoolwork. His family describes him as bright and motivated but notes his difficulty keeping up with peers despite putting in extra effort.

Key Symptoms:

- **Academic Challenges in Reading and Math**: Liam shows marked difficulty with reading fluency, often misreading words and needing frequent pauses. He struggles with decoding words and has difficulty understanding passages. In math, he has trouble with basic arithmetic, often making simple mistakes in addition and subtraction, and struggles with problem-solving tasks.

- **Emotional Impact and Frustration**: Liam experiences frustration and anxiety around schoolwork. His parents report that he often expresses feelings of inadequacy and fears of not being "smart enough." These feelings sometimes lead him to avoid tasks that involve reading or math.

- **Social and Classroom Behavior**: Although generally well-behaved, Liam occasionally becomes restless and disengaged during reading and math lessons. His teachers have noticed that he tends to give up quickly on tasks he finds challenging, which affects his participation in group activities and class assignments.

Symptom Evolution:

Liam's academic difficulties first became apparent in first grade when he struggled to learn to read at the same pace as his classmates. Despite additional tutoring, his reading and math skills remained behind grade level. As the academic demands increased, his challenges became more pronounced, especially in areas requiring complex reading comprehension and math reasoning.

Previous Interventions or Diagnoses:

Liam's school provided additional support through reading and math tutoring, but despite these efforts, he continues to struggle. His parents sought an evaluation from the school psychologist, who suggested the possibility of a learning disorder and recommended further testing.

Clinical Decision-Making Process

DSM-5-TR Diagnostic Criteria Considered:
- **Specific Learning Disorder Criteria**: Liam meets the DSM-5-TR criteria for Specific Learning Disorder, which requires difficulties in learning and using academic skills that persist despite targeted intervention. His reading and math struggles are significantly below age expectations and are not attributable to intellectual disabilities, sensory deficits, or lack of educational opportunity.

- **Domains and Areas Affected**: Liam's primary areas of difficulty fall within the domains of reading (specifically reading fluency and comprehension) and mathematics (basic arithmetic and problem-solving). These persistent academic challenges significantly impact his daily functioning in school.

Exclusion of Other Diagnoses:
- **Intellectual Disability**: Liam's overall cognitive abilities are age-appropriate, and his difficulties are specific to reading and math, which is consistent with Specific Learning Disorder rather than a general intellectual impairment.

- **Attention-Deficit/Hyperactivity Disorder (ADHD)**: Although Liam displays signs of frustration and disengagement, his behavior is specifically related to academic tasks he finds challenging, rather than pervasive attention deficits. ADHD was considered but ruled out based on this task-specific pattern.

- **Anxiety Disorder**: While Liam shows signs of school-related anxiety, this is viewed as secondary to his academic difficulties rather than a primary diagnosis. His anxiety appears to be a response to his learning challenges rather than a standalone disorder.

Assessment Tools:
- **Wechsler Individual Achievement Test (WIAT-III)**: This test assessed Liam's abilities in various academic areas, highlighting significant deficits in reading fluency, reading comprehension, and basic arithmetic. His scores in these areas were well below age and grade expectations, supporting a diagnosis of Specific Learning Disorder.

- **Woodcock-Johnson IV Tests of Achievement**: Used to further evaluate Liam's specific academic skills, this assessment confirmed his struggles with decoding, reading comprehension, and math fluency.

- **Behavior Assessment System for Children (BASC-3)**: Completed by both parents and teachers, this tool provided additional insight into Liam's emotional response to academic challenges, highlighting school-related frustration and anxiety, which further informed the diagnosis and the need for supportive interventions.

Family Discussion: The clinician met with Liam's parents to discuss the diagnosis and explain how a Specific Learning Disorder differs from general academic struggles. The importance of targeted interventions, such as specialized tutoring and accommodations in the classroom, was emphasized. The clinician also discussed potential strategies to manage Liam's anxiety and build his confidence, helping his parents understand the value of creating a supportive, low-stress learning environment at home.

Suggested Topics
- Overview of Specific Learning Disorder and its subtypes (e.g., dyslexia, dyscalculia).
- Understanding and using academic assessment tools, such as WIAT-III and Woodcock-Johnson IV.
- Classroom and home-based strategies for supporting children with Specific Learning Disorder.

Chapter 14: **Clinical Cases in Schizophrenia and Other Psychotic Disorders**

14.0 Introduction to Psychotic Disorders

Psychotic disorders encompass a range of mental health conditions characterized by disruptions in perception, thought processes, emotions, and behaviors. These disorders often involve significant impairments in a person's ability to discern reality, leading to symptoms such as delusions, hallucinations, disorganized thinking, and abnormal motor behaviors. The DSM-5-TR classifies psychotic disorders into distinct categories based on symptom duration, symptom patterns, and the presence of mood disturbances, yet these disorders frequently overlap in presentation, requiring a nuanced approach to diagnosis.

Psychotic disorders typically emerge in late adolescence or early adulthood, with conditions such as schizophrenia manifesting gradually and often requiring lifelong management. Early symptoms, including social withdrawal, flat affect, and cognitive impairments, can make initial identification challenging, especially as these signs often precede full-blown psychotic episodes. The complexity of psychotic disorders is further amplified by factors such as genetic predisposition, environmental influences, and comorbid conditions, including mood disorders and substance use, which can both exacerbate and obscure symptoms.

Effective diagnosis relies on a comprehensive evaluation, using DSM-5-TR criteria to distinguish between similar presentations, such as differentiating schizophrenia from schizoaffective disorder or brief psychotic disorder. Clinicians must assess symptom type, frequency, and severity, as well as the duration of psychotic episodes and any associated mood symptoms. Tools such as structured interviews, symptom rating scales, and consultations with family members play a vital role in accurately identifying these conditions and developing an appropriate treatment plan.

This chapter presents a range of real-world clinical cases to illustrate the diagnostic processes, therapeutic strategies, and long-term management considerations unique to psychotic disorders. By examining these cases, clinicians and students can gain insights into the complexities of diagnosis, explore the differential diagnostic pathways, and appreciate the importance of integrated treatment approaches that encompass medication, therapy, and psychosocial support.

Case 14.1: Schizophrenia

Patient Presentation

Patient: Alex, a 23-year-old male

Family Background: Alex lives with his parents in a suburban area. His family describes him as a once outgoing and creative young man who enjoyed art and music but has become increasingly withdrawn over the past year. He has limited social connections outside of his family, having distanced himself from friends. His parents have grown concerned about his increasingly strange behavior and declining self-care.

Key Symptoms:
- **Positive Symptoms**: Alex reports hearing voices that are not present, often calling him by name and commenting on his actions. He has also developed delusional beliefs, including the idea that he is under surveillance by "unknown entities" and that he possesses a special ability to communicate telepathically. These symptoms cause significant distress and interfere with his daily activities.

- **Negative Symptoms**: Alex displays a marked reduction in emotional expression, often appearing unresponsive or indifferent in social settings. He speaks in a monotone voice, shows little facial expression, and avoids eye contact. He has also shown a diminished interest in previously enjoyed activities.

- **Cognitive Impairments**: He struggles with concentration, often getting distracted during conversations, and has difficulty completing tasks. His parents report that he has been neglecting basic hygiene and personal care, such as showering and changing clothes.

Symptom Evolution:

Alex's symptoms began insidiously around age 21, with early signs including social withdrawal, reduced interest in hobbies, and a noticeable decline in academic performance during his college years. Over the past year, his condition has worsened, with auditory hallucinations and paranoid delusions becoming more frequent and impairing his ability to function. His family initially attributed his behaviors to stress, but as his symptoms persisted and intensified, they sought psychiatric assistance.

Previous Interventions or Diagnoses:

Alex has no formal previous diagnoses but attended a counseling session at his college, where he briefly discussed feeling "different" and "monitored." The counselor recommended a psychiatric evaluation, but he discontinued sessions before further assessment. His family now seeks a comprehensive evaluation to understand his recent behavior and mental health challenges.

Clinical Decision-Making Process

DSM-5-TR Diagnostic Criteria Considered:
- **Criterion A: Key Symptoms**: Alex demonstrates multiple key symptoms of schizophrenia, including auditory hallucinations, delusions of reference, and disorganized thinking, which are consistent with DSM-5-TR criteria for schizophrenia.

- **Duration**: His symptoms have persisted for over six months, with a noticeable decline in social and occupational functioning, fulfilling the criterion of duration for a schizophrenia diagnosis.

- **Functional Impairment**: Alex's delusions, hallucinations, and negative symptoms (e.g., flat affect, social withdrawal) have significantly impacted his daily life, relationships, and self-care, confirming functional impairment.

Exclusion of Other Diagnoses:
- **Schizoaffective Disorder**: Although Alex shows psychotic symptoms, there is no evidence of concurrent mood episodes (such as major depressive or manic episodes), allowing schizoaffective disorder to be ruled out.

- **Substance/Medication-Induced Psychotic Disorder**: Alex's symptoms do not appear to be the result of substance use or withdrawal. His family confirmed no recent history of drug or alcohol use, and a toxicology screen was negative, supporting the exclusion of substance-induced psychosis.

- **Brief Psychotic Disorder**: Due to the chronicity and persistence of symptoms, brief psychotic disorder is ruled out, as it is characterized by episodes lasting less than one month.

Assessment Tools:
- **Positive and Negative Syndrome Scale (PANSS)**: This scale was used to assess the severity of Alex's positive, negative, and general psychopathology symptoms. PANSS results highlighted pronounced positive symptoms (hallucinations, delusions) and significant negative symptoms (flat affect, social withdrawal).

- **Structured Clinical Interview for DSM-5 Disorders (SCID-5)**: This semi-structured interview helped confirm the presence of key schizophrenia symptoms and provided additional insight into Alex's mental state, supporting the diagnosis.

- **Cognitive Assessment (e.g., Trail Making Test, Stroop Test)**: These assessments revealed cognitive impairments in executive functioning, memory, and attention, common in schizophrenia, which further validated the diagnosis.

Family Discussion: The clinician held a session with Alex's parents to explain the nature of schizophrenia, including typical symptom progression and treatment options. The clinician discussed the benefits of antipsychotic medication and supportive therapy, as well as the role of family support in managing the disorder. Emphasis was placed on understanding schizophrenia as a chronic condition with potential for symptom management and improvement with appropriate treatment. This discussion helped Alex's family understand his behaviors within the context of mental illness and provided guidance on ways to support him effectively.

Suggested Topics
- Overview of positive, negative, and cognitive symptoms in schizophrenia.
- Understanding the role of antipsychotic medications and their mechanisms.
- Cognitive impairments associated with schizophrenia and strategies for support.
- Family support strategies for individuals with schizophrenia.

Case 14.2: Schizoaffective Disorder

Patient Presentation
Patient: Maria, a 28-year-old female

Family Background: Maria lives alone and works part-time as a graphic designer. She has a close relationship with her parents and two siblings, who have expressed growing concern over her behavior and emotional health. Her family reports that she has always been sensitive and occasionally moody, but recent behaviors and emotional swings have been more pronounced and disruptive.

Key Symptoms:
- **Mood Symptoms**: Maria experiences cycles of depressive and manic episodes, characterized by periods of severe sadness, low energy, and loss of interest in daily activities, alternating with episodes of elevated mood, decreased need for sleep, increased energy, and impulsive decision-making. These mood disturbances significantly interfere with her ability to maintain stable employment and relationships.

- **Psychotic Symptoms**: During both mood episodes and neutral periods, Maria reports auditory hallucinations, often hearing voices that comment on her actions or make derogatory remarks. She also exhibits paranoid delusions, believing that her coworkers are conspiring against her or monitoring her every move. These symptoms persist regardless of her mood state.

- **Cognitive and Social Impairment**: Maria displays occasional disorganized thinking, evident in her tangential speech patterns and difficulty following conversations. Socially, she has become increasingly isolated, often canceling plans and expressing fear of being judged or ridiculed by others.

Symptom Evolution:

Maria's symptoms began to emerge in her early twenties with mood swings and periods of low energy and depressive thoughts. By age 25, she began to experience auditory hallucinations and delusional thinking during both depressive and elevated mood states. Over time, her condition has worsened, with mood episodes and psychotic symptoms persisting despite attempts to manage stress and lifestyle changes.

Previous Interventions or Diagnoses:

Maria was initially diagnosed with Major Depressive Disorder and was treated with antidepressants. However, her condition did not improve, and she later sought help from a psychiatrist, who noted signs of hypomanic episodes and prescribed a mood stabilizer. With continued symptoms of hallucinations and delusions, Maria was referred for a more comprehensive evaluation to determine an accurate diagnosis.

Clinical Decision-Making Process

DSM-5-TR Diagnostic Criteria Considered:
- **Concurrent Mood and Psychotic Symptoms**: Maria experiences psychotic symptoms, such as hallucinations and delusions, that persist in both depressive and manic states. These symptoms fulfill the DSM-5-TR criteria for schizoaffective disorder, which requires both psychotic symptoms and major mood episodes.

- **Duration of Psychotic Symptoms Independent of Mood Episodes**: Schizoaffective disorder requires that psychotic symptoms, such as hallucinations or delusions, continue for at least two weeks in the absence of any major mood episode. Maria's psychotic symptoms, particularly auditory hallucinations and paranoid delusions, have been present during neutral mood states as well, supporting this criterion.

Exclusion of Other Diagnoses:
- **Bipolar I Disorder with Psychotic Features**: Although Maria has mood episodes and psychotic symptoms, the persistence of her hallucinations and delusions outside of mood episodes differentiates her condition from Bipolar I Disorder with Psychotic Features.

- **Schizophrenia**: While Maria experiences psychotic symptoms, her concurrent mood disturbances, particularly the distinct cycles of depressive and manic episodes, indicate schizoaffective disorder rather than schizophrenia.

- **Major Depressive Disorder with Psychotic Features**: Maria's manic symptoms rule out a diagnosis of Major Depressive Disorder, as she meets the criteria for mood episodes characteristic of bipolar-type schizoaffective disorder.

Assessment Tools:
- **Structured Clinical Interview for DSM-5 Disorders (SCID-5)**: This tool was used to gather comprehensive information on Maria's symptoms, clarifying her psychotic and mood symptoms and providing a structured framework to confirm the presence of schizoaffective disorder.

- **Young Mania Rating Scale (YMRS)** and **Hamilton Depression Rating Scale (HDRS)**: These scales were administered to assess the severity of her manic and depressive symptoms, confirming the cyclical nature of her mood disturbances.

- **Positive and Negative Syndrome Scale (PANSS)**: Used to evaluate Maria's psychotic symptoms, this scale provided insight into her hallucinations, delusions, and disorganized thinking, supporting the diagnosis of schizoaffective disorder with prominent psychotic features.

Family Discussion: The clinician involved Maria's family in the diagnostic process, providing an explanation of schizoaffective disorder and how it differs from schizophrenia and bipolar disorder. Emphasis was placed on the importance of ongoing mood stabilization and antipsychotic treatment, as well as supportive therapy. The family was encouraged to maintain open communication with Maria and to recognize potential warning signs of mood or psychotic episodes. This conversation helped clarify Maria's diagnosis for her family and provided them with tools to better support her.

Suggested Topics
- Differentiating Schizoaffective Disorder from Bipolar Disorder with Psychotic Features.
- Overview of mood-stabilizing and antipsychotic medications in managing schizoaffective disorder.
- Role of family support and psychoeducation in the treatment of schizoaffective disorder.

Case 14.3: Brief Psychotic Disorder

Patient Presentation
Patient: Daniel, a 30-year-old male

Family Background: Daniel is single and lives alone in a busy metropolitan area. He works as a software developer and generally has a high-stress work environment. His family describes him as responsible, grounded, and calm, with no prior history of mental health issues. Recently, Daniel's friends and family were shocked by an unexpected episode of unusual behavior and paranoia that seemed out of character.

Key Symptoms:
- **Sudden Onset of Psychotic Symptoms**: Daniel experienced a sudden onset of psychotic symptoms, including auditory hallucinations in which he heard a voice commanding him to "take action" against imaginary enemies. He also displayed paranoid delusions, believing that his coworkers were plotting to sabotage his work and ruin his career.
- **Disorganized Behavior**: During the episode, Daniel displayed disorganized behavior, such as talking to himself, pacing around his apartment, and becoming increasingly agitated. He seemed unable to focus on his daily activities, and his hygiene and self-care rapidly deteriorated within a short period.
- **Duration of Episode**: His symptoms began abruptly after a high-stress week at work and lasted for approximately one week. The symptoms gradually subsided with supportive care and rest, with Daniel returning to his baseline functioning soon after.

Symptom Evolution:

Daniel had never previously exhibited any symptoms of psychosis or other mental health issues. The psychotic episode appeared to emerge spontaneously following a period of intense stress at work, accompanied by several nights of inadequate sleep. His family reported that, following this period of stress, Daniel became withdrawn and expressed strange ideas. Over the course of one week, his symptoms peaked with intense paranoia, hallucinations, and erratic behavior, but they began to subside with minimal intervention, eventually disappearing entirely by the end of the week.

Previous Interventions or Diagnoses:

Daniel had no prior mental health diagnoses or treatments. His family initially sought help when they observed his abrupt change in behavior, and he was taken to an emergency psychiatric evaluation during the peak of his symptoms. There, he received supportive care, and his symptoms resolved without pharmacological treatment.

Clinical Decision-Making Process

DSM-5-TR Diagnostic Criteria Considered:
- **Presence of One or More Key Psychotic Symptoms**: Daniel exhibited both hallucinations (auditory) and delusions (paranoia), fulfilling the DSM-5-TR requirement for brief psychotic disorder.

- **Duration of Symptoms**: The symptoms lasted for less than one month (approximately one week), which meets the DSM-5-TR criteria for brief psychotic disorder.

- **Return to Baseline Functioning**: After the resolution of the psychotic symptoms, Daniel returned to his typical level of functioning, with no residual symptoms, further supporting a diagnosis of brief psychotic disorder.

Exclusion of Other Diagnoses:
- **Schizophrenia**: Schizophrenia was ruled out due to the brief duration of symptoms and the absence of a longer history of psychotic episodes or functional decline.

- **Schizophreniform Disorder**: Although Daniel experienced acute psychotic symptoms, the brief duration of less than one month differentiates brief psychotic disorder from schizophreniform disorder, which requires a symptom duration of at least one month but less than six months.
- **Substance-Induced Psychotic Disorder**: Toxicology screenings during the evaluation revealed no evidence of substance use or intoxication, ruling out a substance-induced psychotic episode.

Assessment Tools:
- **Mental Status Examination (MSE)**: Conducted during his emergency evaluation, the MSE confirmed the presence of auditory hallucinations, paranoid delusions, and disorganized thought processes, supporting the brief psychotic episode diagnosis.

- **Clinical Interview and Family History**: The clinical interview provided information on Daniel's psychosocial background, recent stressors, and lack of previous psychiatric symptoms, reinforcing the likelihood of a stress-induced brief psychotic disorder.

- **Brief Psychiatric Rating Scale (BPRS)**: Used to quantify the severity of his symptoms during the episode, this assessment confirmed significant but transient psychotic symptoms. The BPRS was administered again post-episode, demonstrating a complete return to baseline.

Family Discussion: The clinician held a session with Daniel and his family to explain the nature of brief psychotic disorder, emphasizing that such episodes can occur in response to extreme stress, often resolving completely after the stressor is mitigated. The clinician discussed potential coping mechanisms, stress management techniques, and advised family members on early warning signs to monitor in case of recurrence. This helped reassure the family and provided Daniel with strategies to manage future stress.

Suggested Topics
- Understanding the role of acute stress in triggering brief psychotic disorder.
- Differential diagnosis between brief psychotic disorder, schizophreniform disorder, and schizophrenia.
- Stress management and coping strategies to prevent future episodes of brief psychotic disorder.

Case 14.4: Delusional Disorder

Patient Presentation

Patient: Laura, a 45-year-old female

Family Background: Laura is a single woman living independently. She works as a receptionist at a law firm and is known for her attention to detail and professionalism. Over the past year, her family and coworkers have noticed an increasing preoccupation with a specific belief that appears irrational to them, yet she remains otherwise well-functioning. Her family describes her as highly organized and private, with few close friends or social activities outside of work.

Key Symptoms:

- **Delusional Beliefs**: Laura holds a fixed delusion that she is under surveillance by a group of unknown individuals attempting to sabotage her professional reputation. She believes that these individuals follow her to work, manipulate her work environment, and spread rumors about her within the community. Despite reassurance from family and coworkers, Laura remains convinced of the surveillance and frequently changes her daily routes or routines to "evade" these individuals.

- **Lack of Hallucinations**: Laura has no history of auditory or visual hallucinations, nor does she experience any disorganized thinking, behaviors, or cognitive impairments outside of her delusional belief.

- **Preserved Social and Occupational Functioning**: Laura's belief in the surveillance affects her daily life in specific ways—she has become more withdrawn and has developed some mistrust toward her coworkers—but she continues to perform her job duties effectively. Her social interactions are otherwise appropriate, and she exhibits no bizarre behavior beyond her delusion.

Symptom Evolution:

Laura's delusional beliefs emerged gradually over the past year, beginning with subtle suspicions about her workplace. Over time, her beliefs intensified, and she became increasingly preoccupied with her conviction of being watched. This preoccupation has caused some strain in her relationships, as she frequently seeks reassurance from her family and responds defensively when they question her beliefs.

Previous Interventions or Diagnoses:

Laura has no history of psychiatric diagnoses or treatment. She sought initial counseling after her family urged her to address her suspicions, but she discontinued after a few sessions, feeling that the therapist did not "take her concerns seriously." She reluctantly agreed to another evaluation when her family expressed ongoing concern.

Clinical Decision-Making Process

DSM-5-TR Diagnostic Criteria Considered:
- **Presence of One or More Delusions**: Laura meets the DSM-5-TR criteria for delusional disorder, having a single, well-defined delusion of being surveilled and targeted. Her belief is not considered bizarre, as it involves a plausible, though false, scenario of surveillance.

- **Duration**: Her delusional belief has persisted for over one year, fulfilling the DSM-5-TR criterion for duration in delusional disorder.

- **Lack of Other Psychotic Symptoms**: Laura does not display hallucinations, disorganized speech, or behavior. Her cognitive abilities and overall functioning are preserved outside of the influence of her delusion.

Exclusion of Other Diagnoses:
- **Schizophrenia**: Laura does not meet the criteria for schizophrenia, as she lacks additional psychotic symptoms, such as hallucinations or disorganized thinking, and her delusion is isolated and fixed rather than part of a broader psychotic syndrome.

- **Obsessive-Compulsive Disorder (OCD)**: While Laura exhibits repetitive checking behaviors, these actions stem directly from her delusion rather than from intrusive obsessive thoughts, which distinguishes her case from OCD.

- **Mood Disorder with Psychotic Features**: Laura does not exhibit depressive or manic symptoms that would suggest a mood disorder with psychotic features, and her delusional belief is not accompanied by mood dysregulation.

Assessment Tools:
- **Structured Clinical Interview for DSM-5 Disorders (SCID-5)**: This tool was used to confirm the presence of Laura's delusional belief, verifying the duration and impact on her life, and ruling out other psychotic or mood symptoms.

- **Beck Depression Inventory (BDI)**: Administered to assess whether mood disturbances might be influencing her thoughts. Laura's results were within the normal range, supporting the exclusion of mood-related psychotic features.

- **Yale-Brown Obsessive Compulsive Scale (Y-BOCS)**: Used to differentiate her repetitive checking from obsessions or compulsions, which are characteristic of OCD. Her checking behavior was found to be directly tied to her delusional beliefs rather than intrusive thoughts.

Family Discussion: The clinician met with Laura's family to discuss delusional disorder, explaining how it differs from other psychotic disorders and providing guidance on how to support Laura without reinforcing her delusions. The family was encouraged to avoid direct confrontation of her beliefs, which could heighten defensiveness, and instead to focus on maintaining open and supportive communication. The clinician also discussed the potential benefits of psychotherapy for Laura, specifically cognitive-behavioral approaches that may help her examine and possibly reduce the intensity of her beliefs.

Suggested Topics
- Overview of delusional disorder subtypes and differential diagnosis.
- Cognitive-behavioral therapy approaches for delusional disorder.
- Family support strategies for individuals with delusional disorder.

Case 14.5: Catatonia

Patient Presentation

Patient: Brian, a 32-year-old male

Family Background: Brian lives with his parents and has a close relationship with his two younger siblings. He has a history of major depressive disorder, for which he has received intermittent treatment over the years. Recently, his family has been concerned about his sudden withdrawal and changes in behavior. His mother reports that over the past two weeks, he has become largely unresponsive and often remains motionless for extended periods.

Key Symptoms:

- **Catatonic Stupor and Mutism**: Brian exhibits a profound lack of responsiveness to his surroundings. He spends hours sitting or lying motionless, staring blankly, and does not respond verbally or physically to attempts at interaction.

- **Posturing and Negativism**: He frequently adopts rigid postures and resists movement or attempts to adjust his position. His family notes that he resists attempts to help him eat or move, and at times seems to actively oppose any effort to engage him.

- **Stereotypy and Mannerisms**: Occasionally, Brian displays repetitive, purposeless movements such as rocking or repetitive hand gestures. His family reports that these behaviors appear spontaneous and unrelated to his environment.

Symptom Evolution:

Brian's symptoms appeared abruptly following a particularly stressful period at work, where he experienced increased depressive symptoms, including low energy, feelings of hopelessness, and difficulty concentrating. After several weeks of intensified depressive symptoms, his behavior became increasingly withdrawn, and within days he was exhibiting catatonic signs. His family initially assumed he was dealing with heightened depression, but his symptoms rapidly worsened, leading them to seek immediate medical assistance.

Previous Interventions or Diagnoses:

Brian was diagnosed with major depressive disorder five years ago and has received treatment with antidepressants intermittently. Although his depressive episodes were sometimes severe, he had not previously exhibited psychotic or catatonic symptoms. His history of depression and recent stress raised concerns about a potential worsening of his condition.

Clinical Decision-Making Process

DSM-5-TR Diagnostic Criteria Considered:
- **Presence of Catatonic Features**: According to DSM-5-TR, catatonia is diagnosed when three or more of the following symptoms are present: stupor, mutism, negativism, posturing, and stereotypy. Brian meets these criteria, displaying stupor, mutism, posturing, negativism, and stereotypy, confirming the presence of catatonia.
- **Context and Associated Condition**: Catatonia can be associated with several mental health conditions, including mood disorders, psychotic disorders, or as a stand-alone diagnosis. Given Brian's history of major depressive disorder, his catatonic symptoms are likely secondary to a severe depressive episode.

Exclusion of Other Diagnoses:
- **Schizophrenia**: While catatonia can occur in schizophrenia, Brian has no history of schizophrenia-related symptoms such as delusions or hallucinations. His symptoms are better explained by his history of major depressive disorder.

- **Neurological or Medical Conditions**: To rule out medical causes, Brian underwent a comprehensive medical evaluation, including neurological exams and brain imaging, which returned normal results. This ruled out medical causes such as seizure disorders or metabolic imbalances.

- **Substance-Induced Catatonia**: Toxicology screenings were negative, ruling out catatonia induced by substance use or medication side effects.

Assessment Tools:
- **Bush-Francis Catatonia Rating Scale (BFCRS)**: This scale was used to assess the severity of Brian's catatonic symptoms, confirming the presence of stupor, mutism, and posturing. The BFCRS score supported a diagnosis of catatonia due to the severity and pervasiveness of his symptoms.

- **Structured Clinical Interview for DSM-5 Disorders (SCID-5)**: This interview confirmed the persistence of depressive symptoms and provided a structured assessment of Brian's mental health history, clarifying the association between his catatonic symptoms and his pre-existing depressive disorder.

- **Comprehensive Medical Evaluation**: Additional lab tests and imaging ruled out metabolic, neurological, or systemic causes, reinforcing the conclusion that Brian's catatonic state is psychiatric in origin.

Family Discussion: The clinician met with Brian's family to discuss the diagnosis of catatonia and its potential link to his depressive disorder. The family was provided with information on the nature of catatonia and its treatment options, including the use of benzodiazepines, which are often effective in reducing catatonic symptoms. The clinician explained the importance of hospitalization to provide Brian with supervised care and monitor his response to treatment, which helped the family understand the urgency and necessity of immediate intervention.

Suggested Topics
- Understanding catatonia and its subtypes.
- Pharmacological interventions for catatonia, including benzodiazepine use.
- Differential diagnosis: distinguishing catatonia from neurological and medical conditions.

Chapter 15: Clinical Cases in Bipolar and Related Disorders

Introduction to Bipolar and Related Disorders

Bipolar and related disorders encompass a spectrum of mood disorders characterized by significant fluctuations in mood, energy levels, and activity. These conditions are marked by periods of intense emotional states—referred to as mood episodes—which vary between manic, hypomanic, and depressive phases. While mood episodes differ in severity and duration across the bipolar spectrum, the hallmark of bipolar disorders is the occurrence of manic or hypomanic episodes, which distinguish them from depressive disorders.

Bipolar I Disorder, defined by the presence of at least one full manic episode, represents the most severe form of bipolar disorder and can include major depressive episodes. Bipolar II Disorder, by contrast, involves episodes of hypomania—less intense than full mania—and major depressive episodes, often leading to significant impairment even though manic symptoms are milder. Cyclothymic Disorder is characterized by chronic mood fluctuations that do not meet the full criteria for hypomanic or depressive episodes, resulting in persistent mood instability. Additionally, substance/medication-induced bipolar disorder may occur when mood disturbances are directly linked to substance use or withdrawal, highlighting the interplay between external factors and mood dysregulation.

In clinical practice, diagnosing bipolar and related disorders requires careful assessment to differentiate between manic, hypomanic, and depressive episodes, as well as to recognize mixed features, rapid cycling, and comorbid conditions that may complicate the presentation. Accurate diagnosis is critical, as bipolar disorders can be misdiagnosed as major depressive disorder if manic or hypomanic symptoms go unreported or unnoticed. Pharmacological treatment, typically involving mood stabilizers, antipsychotics, and antidepressants (with caution), is essential for managing mood episodes and preventing recurrence. Psychotherapy, psychoeducation, and lifestyle modifications also play vital roles in helping individuals and families cope with the complexities of these disorders.

This chapter provides a series of clinical cases to illustrate the diversity within bipolar and related disorders. Through these real-world examples, clinicians and students can explore the diagnostic challenges and treatment considerations unique to each condition, gaining a deeper understanding of effective approaches to managing bipolar disorder and supporting long-term patient wellness.

Case 15.1: Bipolar I Disorder

Patient Presentation
Patient: David, a 27-year-old male

Family Background: David lives with his wife and 3-year-old daughter in a suburban neighborhood. He works as a project manager in a high-demand technology firm. His family describes him as energetic, driven, and highly social. Over the past few months, however, his behavior has become erratic, and his family has grown increasingly concerned about his well-being. He has no significant prior psychiatric history but has struggled with stress-related symptoms intermittently.

Key Symptoms:
- **Manic Episode**: David recently exhibited classic manic symptoms, including increased energy, reduced need for sleep (sleeping only 2-3 hours per night without feeling tired), racing thoughts, and pressured speech. He has been engaging in impulsive behaviors, such as excessive spending on luxury items and initiating risky business ventures without discussing them with his wife.

- **Grandiosity and Inflated Self-Esteem**: He expressed grandiose ideas, believing that he had discovered a revolutionary business concept that would "transform the industry" and frequently proclaimed he was "destined for greatness."

- **Increased Irritability and Impulsivity**: David displayed irritability when his wife questioned his decisions, becoming defensive and dismissive of her concerns. He also engaged in risky behaviors, such as excessive alcohol consumption and impulsive travel arrangements without informing his family.

Symptom Evolution:

David's symptoms appeared gradually but intensified over the course of two weeks. Initially, his wife noticed he was staying up late and seemed more enthusiastic about work, which was uncharacteristic. Over the next few days, he became noticeably more excitable, talkative, and distracted, eventually exhibiting behavior that alarmed his family. His impulsive spending and risky business ventures began to strain the family's finances and relationships. This episode has been his first experience with severe manic symptoms.

Previous Interventions or Diagnoses:

David has no formal history of mood disorders. He experienced stress-related symptoms in the past, such as mild insomnia and anxiety during high-pressure work periods, but he has not previously sought mental health treatment. His recent behaviors prompted his family to arrange a psychiatric evaluation.

Clinical Decision-Making Process

DSM-5-TR Diagnostic Criteria Considered:
- **Presence of a Manic Episode**: According to the DSM-5-TR, a diagnosis of Bipolar I Disorder requires at least one manic episode, characterized by a distinct period of abnormally elevated or irritable mood and increased energy lasting at least one week. David's episode of manic symptoms, including decreased need for sleep, grandiosity, and impulsive behaviors, meets these criteria.

- **Functional Impairment**: The impact of his manic symptoms on his work performance, relationships, and financial stability confirms the presence of significant functional impairment, supporting the diagnosis of Bipolar I Disorder.

- **Exclusion of Substance-Induced Mania**: David's toxicology screen was negative, ruling out the possibility that his manic symptoms were caused by substance use or medication.

Exclusion of Other Diagnoses:
- **Bipolar II Disorder**: Bipolar II Disorder was ruled out because it requires the presence of hypomanic episodes rather than full manic episodes, which are less severe and do not cause significant impairment. David's symptoms, including grandiosity and impulsivity, clearly meet the threshold for mania.

- **Cyclothymic Disorder**: Cyclothymic Disorder is characterized by chronic mood fluctuations without meeting full criteria for manic or depressive episodes. David's clear manic episode exceeds the criteria for cyclothymic disorder.

- **Borderline Personality Disorder (BPD)**: Although David exhibits impulsivity and interpersonal difficulties, his symptoms are episodic rather than chronic, occurring specifically during a manic episode. His condition is thus more consistent with Bipolar I Disorder.

Assessment Tools:
- **Young Mania Rating Scale (YMRS)**: This tool assessed the severity of David's manic symptoms, including mood elevation, irritability, sleep disruption, and thought disorder. His scores were consistent with a manic episode, supporting the diagnosis.

- **Mood Disorder Questionnaire (MDQ)**: Used to screen for bipolar disorder, the MDQ provided insight into David's mood symptoms and history. His responses suggested that this was likely his first manic episode, with no history of depressive episodes.

- **Structured Clinical Interview for DSM-5 Disorders (SCID-5)**: This structured interview provided a comprehensive assessment of David's symptom history and helped rule out differential diagnoses. It confirmed his symptoms met the criteria for Bipolar I Disorder.

Family Discussion: The clinician held a session with David and his wife to explain Bipolar I Disorder, focusing on the nature of manic episodes and their potential impact on relationships and daily life. The clinician discussed treatment options, including mood stabilizers, antipsychotic medications, and the role of lifestyle adjustments in managing symptoms. The importance of recognizing early warning signs and establishing a strong support network was emphasized, providing David and his family with tools to prevent or minimize future episodes.

Suggested Topics
- Understanding the difference between manic, hypomanic, and depressive episodes in bipolar disorder.
- Overview of pharmacological treatments for Bipolar I Disorder, including mood stabilizers and antipsychotics.
- Family support strategies and the role of psychoeducation in managing bipolar disorder.

Case 15.2: Bipolar II Disorder

Patient Presentation
Patient: Julia, a 34-year-old female

Family Background: Julia lives with her partner and works as an elementary school teacher. Known to be empathetic and dedicated to her job, she has recently struggled with mood swings that have begun affecting her work performance and relationships. Julia describes herself as having always been "emotional," but recent changes in her mood and behavior have concerned both her and her partner, prompting her to seek help.

Key Symptoms:
- **Depressive Episodes**: Julia has experienced multiple episodes of severe depression over the past several years, each lasting from a few weeks to several months. During these periods, she reports feeling hopeless, experiencing low energy, and losing interest in activities she previously enjoyed. Her concentration and motivation decline significantly, affecting her ability to manage classroom tasks and interact with her students.

- **Hypomanic Episodes**: Between depressive episodes, Julia has periods of heightened energy and mood that last several days. During these hypomanic episodes, she feels more creative and productive, often staying up late to work on lesson plans or engaging in spontaneous projects. However, her partner has noticed that during these times, she is more irritable and prone to impulsive decisions, such as spending excessively on classroom supplies or impulsively planning weekend trips without considering her financial situation.

- **Social Impact**: Julia's depressive episodes have strained her relationship, as she becomes withdrawn and avoids social interaction. During hypomanic periods, her behavior becomes unpredictable, which occasionally leads to conflicts with her partner.

Symptom Evolution:

Julia's symptoms emerged in her late twenties, with depressive episodes occurring periodically. Over the past two years, she has noticed the appearance of hypomanic episodes in addition to her depressive phases. The cycle of mood swings has become more pronounced, with her hypomanic episodes often preceding a depressive period. Her partner urged her to seek help after noticing the patterns and their effect on her professional and personal life.

Previous Interventions or Diagnoses:

Julia was previously diagnosed with Major Depressive Disorder and received treatment with antidepressants, which seemed to alleviate her depressive symptoms but occasionally triggered periods of heightened energy. She discontinued treatment after experiencing mood swings that her previous clinician did not fully address, leading to the current evaluation for a more accurate diagnosis.

Clinical Decision-Making Process

DSM-5-TR Diagnostic Criteria Considered:
- **Presence of Major Depressive Episodes**: Julia meets the DSM-5-TR criteria for major depressive episodes, characterized by persistent low mood, anhedonia, fatigue, and concentration issues, which have occurred repeatedly over the years.

- **Presence of Hypomanic Episodes**: Julia's hypomanic episodes meet the DSM-5-TR criteria, as they include elevated mood, increased energy, decreased need for sleep, and occasional impulsivity. Her episodes last at least four days but do not result in the severe impairment or psychotic features seen in full manic episodes.

- **Absence of Manic Episodes**: Bipolar II Disorder is differentiated by the absence of full manic episodes. Julia's elevated mood and energy never escalate to the level of mania, supporting a diagnosis of Bipolar II Disorder.

Exclusion of Other Diagnoses:
- **Bipolar I Disorder**: While Julia experiences hypomanic episodes, she has not experienced full manic episodes, differentiating her condition from Bipolar I Disorder.

- **Cyclothymic Disorder**: Cyclothymic Disorder was ruled out due to the presence of distinct major depressive episodes, as cyclothymia involves mood fluctuations without meeting criteria for major depressive or hypomanic episodes.

- **Borderline Personality Disorder (BPD)**: Julia's mood fluctuations are episodic, rather than occurring daily, and her behavior does not exhibit the chronic impulsivity and relational instability typically associated with BPD.

Assessment Tools:
- **Hypomania Checklist-32 (HCL-32)**: This self-report tool helped Julia and her clinician identify symptoms of hypomania, confirming the presence of behaviors and mood changes associated with hypomanic episodes.

- **Hamilton Depression Rating Scale (HDRS)**: Administered to assess the severity of Julia's depressive episodes, the HDRS results were consistent with major depressive episodes, further supporting the diagnosis of Bipolar II Disorder.

- **Structured Clinical Interview for DSM-5 Disorders (SCID-5)**: The SCID-5 provided a comprehensive evaluation of Julia's mood history and excluded other potential diagnoses, confirming the presence of both major depressive and hypomanic episodes without full mania.

Family Discussion: The clinician met with Julia and her partner to discuss the diagnosis of Bipolar II Disorder, emphasizing how hypomanic episodes differ from mania and explaining the impact of these mood swings on her relationships and daily life. They discussed treatment options, including mood stabilizers, to manage both her depressive and hypomanic symptoms. Julia and her partner were educated on identifying early signs of mood shifts and encouraged to communicate openly about her needs and challenges. Psychoeducation on the importance of routine and sleep was also provided to help stabilize her mood.

Suggested Topics
- Understanding the distinction between Bipolar I and Bipolar II Disorder.
- Pharmacological approaches to managing hypomanic and depressive episodes in Bipolar II Disorder.
- Lifestyle strategies and psychoeducation for managing Bipolar II Disorder.

Case 15.3: Cyclothymic Disorder

Patient Presentation
Patient: Tom, a 38-year-old male

Family Background: Tom lives with his long-term partner and works as a freelance writer. Known for his creativity and humor, Tom's family describes him as "moody" and highly sensitive. He has had frequent changes in mood and energy, but his symptoms never seemed severe enough to seek treatment until now. Tom has no previous history of psychiatric treatment, though his partner encouraged him to seek help due to ongoing mood fluctuations that have started impacting their relationship and his work.

Key Symptoms:
- **Chronic Mood Instability**: For at least the past two years, Tom has experienced frequent mood swings ranging from mild depressive states, where he feels low energy and pessimistic, to hypomanic-like periods characterized by increased energy, optimism, and productivity. These mood shifts do not meet the full criteria for either a major depressive episode or a hypomanic episode.

- **Low-Grade Depressive Symptoms**: During his lower mood phases, Tom feels fatigued, unmotivated, and withdrawn. While he doesn't meet full criteria for major depression, he describes these periods as challenging, often resulting in low productivity and social withdrawal.

- **Hypomanic-Like Symptoms**: In his elevated phases, Tom becomes more social, talkative, and energized, often taking on multiple projects. However, his confidence can sometimes lead him to make impulsive decisions, such as accepting unrealistic deadlines. These elevated periods are generally brief and do not cause severe impairment.

- **Minimal Functional Impairment**: While his mood shifts affect his relationship and occasionally his work consistency, he remains functional and has not experienced full-blown manic or depressive episodes that would require hospitalization or disrupt his life entirely.

Symptom Evolution:

Tom's mood swings have been present for as long as he can remember but became more problematic in his mid-thirties. He attributes the worsening symptoms to increased work stress, which seems to intensify both his low and high mood phases. Over the past year, his partner has expressed concern that Tom's moods are unpredictable, making it difficult to plan activities or commitments together. Despite these issues, Tom is hesitant to identify as having a mood disorder, describing his mood changes as "just part of my personality."

Previous Interventions or Diagnoses:

Tom has not sought psychiatric treatment before and has no formal diagnoses. This current evaluation is his first step toward understanding his chronic mood instability, with a focus on determining whether his symptoms align with a specific mood disorder.

Clinical Decision-Making Process

DSM-5-TR Diagnostic Criteria Considered:
- **Chronic Mood Fluctuations**: Cyclothymic disorder is diagnosed when mood fluctuations last for at least two years in adults and include numerous periods of hypomanic and depressive symptoms without meeting full criteria for hypomanic, manic, or major depressive episodes. Tom's long-standing pattern of mild mood elevation and low-grade depressive symptoms over the past two years supports this diagnosis.

- **Absence of Major Mood Episodes**: Tom's symptoms do not meet the full criteria for major depressive or hypomanic episodes, which is consistent with the requirements for cyclothymic disorder.

- **Functional Impact**: While Tom's mood swings impact his personal relationships and work consistency, they do not cause severe impairment or require hospitalization, aligning with the nature of cyclothymic disorder.

Exclusion of Other Diagnoses:
- **Bipolar I and Bipolar II Disorder**: Both were excluded, as Tom's mood fluctuations do not meet the criteria for full manic, hypomanic, or major depressive episodes.

- **Borderline Personality Disorder (BPD)**: Though Tom exhibits mood instability, his symptoms are periodic rather than daily, and he lacks other core features of BPD, such as chronic impulsivity and relationship instability typical of the disorder.

- **Persistent Depressive Disorder (Dysthymia)**: Although Tom experiences low moods, his symptoms alternate between mild depression and mild hypomanic-like states, which are inconsistent with persistent depressive disorder.

Assessment Tools:
- **Mood Disorder Questionnaire (MDQ)**: This self-assessment tool provided insight into Tom's mood fluctuations, ruling out full manic or hypomanic episodes and aligning with the characteristics of cyclothymic disorder.

- **Hypomania Checklist-32 (HCL-32)**: This checklist helped identify the hypomanic-like symptoms present in Tom's mood fluctuations, further supporting a diagnosis of cyclothymic disorder by revealing his chronic, subclinical mood elevation.

- **Beck Depression Inventory (BDI)**: This scale was used to assess the severity of Tom's depressive symptoms. Results indicated mild depressive symptoms that did not meet the threshold for a major depressive episode, supporting a diagnosis of cyclothymic disorder.

Family Discussion: The clinician discussed the diagnosis with Tom and his partner, explaining the chronic but mild nature of cyclothymic disorder and how it differs from other bipolar and mood disorders. The clinician emphasized that mood stabilization strategies, such as cognitive-behavioral therapy (CBT) and lifestyle changes, could help Tom manage his mood swings. Tom and his partner were encouraged to work together to recognize early signs of mood shifts, creating a supportive approach to managing his condition. Psychoeducation on maintaining regular sleep, reducing stress, and limiting alcohol intake was also provided.

Suggested Topics
- Overview of cyclothymic disorder and its differentiation from other bipolar spectrum disorders.
- Lifestyle modifications and the role of psychoeducation in managing cyclothymic disorder.
- Cognitive-behavioral strategies for managing mood instability in cyclothymic disorder.

Case 15.4: Substance/Medication-Induced Bipolar Disorder

Patient Presentation

Patient: Alex, a 40-year-old male

Family Background: Alex lives with his wife and two children in a suburban neighborhood. He works as a pharmacist and is known for being responsible and meticulous in his work. Recently, however, his family and coworkers have noticed changes in his behavior, which have raised concerns. Alex has no prior history of mood disorders, and his family describes him as generally level-headed and calm.

Key Symptoms:
- **Manic Symptoms Induced by Medication**: Over the past two weeks, Alex has exhibited increased energy, reduced need for sleep, and elevated mood. He has become unusually talkative, taking on numerous tasks at work and at home. He also exhibits grandiosity, speaking about starting multiple new business ventures and showing unusual confidence in his abilities. These behaviors are uncharacteristic for him.

- **Impulsivity and Risk-Taking**: Alex has shown impulsive behaviors, such as making large purchases without consulting his wife and neglecting his usual cautious approach. He also became noticeably irritable when his family expressed concerns about his sudden change in behavior.

- **Medication History**: Alex was recently prescribed corticosteroids for a persistent inflammatory condition. His manic-like symptoms appeared shortly after he began this treatment, coinciding with the dosage increase. Alex has no history of psychiatric symptoms prior to starting corticosteroids.

Symptom Evolution:

Alex's behavior changed abruptly, with symptoms emerging within days of increasing his corticosteroid dose. His mood symptoms intensified as the dose was increased, and he has been unable to return to his usual calm and rational self. His family, initially unsure of the cause, suspected a link between his behavior and his new medication regimen, prompting them to seek an evaluation.

Previous Interventions or Diagnoses:

Alex has no prior psychiatric diagnoses. His recent behavioral changes are the first instance of mood dysregulation, which aligns with his recent corticosteroid treatment.

Clinical Decision-Making Process

DSM-5-TR Diagnostic Criteria Considered:
- **Temporal Association with Substance/Medication Use**: According to the DSM-5-TR, Substance/Medication-Induced Bipolar Disorder is diagnosed when mood symptoms emerge during or shortly after substance use or withdrawal, or in association with medication use. Alex's manic symptoms began shortly after starting high-dose corticosteroids, fulfilling this criterion.

- **Presence of Manic Symptoms**: Alex meets the criteria for manic symptoms, including elevated mood, decreased need for sleep, grandiosity, and impulsivity. His symptoms are consistent with a manic episode induced by medication rather than an inherent bipolar disorder.

- **Absence of Prior Mood Episodes**: Alex's lack of prior psychiatric history and the clear link between his symptoms and the corticosteroid treatment support a diagnosis of Substance/Medication-Induced Bipolar Disorder.

Exclusion of Other Diagnoses:
- **Bipolar I Disorder**: Although Alex exhibits symptoms similar to mania, Bipolar I Disorder was ruled out due to the clear temporal relationship between his mood symptoms and his corticosteroid treatment. Additionally, he has no previous history of mood episodes.

- **Cyclothymic Disorder**: Cyclothymic Disorder was ruled out because Alex has no chronic mood instability or history of mood fluctuations. His symptoms appeared suddenly and are directly linked to his medication.

- **Substance-Induced Psychotic Disorder**: Alex's symptoms are mood-related, including grandiosity, impulsivity, and irritability, rather than psychotic in nature. He does not exhibit hallucinations or delusions, which rules out a substance-induced psychotic disorder.

Assessment Tools:
- **Medication History Review**: A detailed medication history was reviewed to determine the onset and escalation of Alex's symptoms, revealing that his mood changes began soon after starting a high dose of corticosteroids.

- **Young Mania Rating Scale (YMRS)**: Used to assess the severity of Alex's manic symptoms, this scale confirmed the presence of clinically significant manic-like symptoms.

- **Clinical Interview**: A structured interview confirmed the temporal link between his corticosteroid use and the onset of symptoms, reinforcing the diagnosis of medication-induced mood disorder. This interview also helped rule out any personal or family history of mood disorders.

Family Discussion: The clinician met with Alex and his family to discuss the diagnosis of Substance/Medication-Induced Bipolar Disorder, explaining the effect of corticosteroids on mood and behavior. The clinician emphasized that the mood symptoms are likely reversible upon adjusting or discontinuing the corticosteroid treatment. Alternatives to corticosteroids were discussed with Alex's prescribing physician to minimize the impact on his mood. His family was advised to monitor his symptoms closely and communicate with his medical team if his behavior changed further.

Suggested Topics
- Mechanisms of mood disturbance associated with corticosteroids and other medications.
- Overview of Substance/Medication-Induced Bipolar Disorder.
- Management strategies for mood stabilization in patients with medication-induced mood disorders.

Case 15.5: Bipolar Disorder with Comorbid Anxiety

Patient Presentation

Patient: Sarah, a 29-year-old female

Family Background: Sarah is married and lives with her husband in an urban area. She works as a graphic designer and is known for her creativity but has struggled with mood swings that impact both her work and her personal life. Recently, Sarah has also been experiencing frequent anxiety symptoms that have intensified her mood episodes and made daily life more challenging. Sarah has a history of Bipolar II Disorder, diagnosed three years ago, and has undergone treatment intermittently.

Key Symptoms:

- **Hypomanic Episodes**: Sarah experiences hypomanic episodes every few months, during which she becomes highly productive, feels "unstoppable," and is able to work for long hours with little sleep. During these episodes, she also exhibits irritability and impatience, especially when others fail to keep up with her rapid pace and ideas.

- **Depressive Episodes**: Between hypomanic episodes, Sarah frequently experiences periods of low mood, characterized by feelings of worthlessness, fatigue, and reduced motivation. She finds it difficult to complete projects, often feeling overwhelmed and experiencing self-doubt about her abilities.

- **Anxiety Symptoms**: Recently, Sarah has started experiencing anxiety symptoms, including persistent worry, restlessness, muscle tension, and episodes of panic, particularly during her depressive phases. The anxiety exacerbates her depressive symptoms, making it harder for her to manage her responsibilities and maintain stable relationships.

Symptom Evolution:

Sarah's bipolar symptoms have been present for several years, but her anxiety symptoms began emerging only recently. Initially, her anxiety manifested as excessive worry about her work performance and relationship stability, but over the past year, it has worsened, contributing to panic attacks and social avoidance. Her anxiety appears to both aggravate and be aggravated by her mood fluctuations, creating a cycle that further destabilizes her mood.

Previous Interventions or Diagnoses:

Sarah has received intermittent treatment for Bipolar II Disorder, including mood stabilizers and antidepressants, but has struggled with medication adherence due to side effects. She has also attended individual therapy periodically. Although anxiety was not initially part of her diagnosis, her recent escalation in symptoms led her therapist to recommend an evaluation for comorbid anxiety.

Clinical Decision-Making Process

DSM-5-TR Diagnostic Criteria Considered:
- **Bipolar II Disorder**: Sarah meets the DSM-5-TR criteria for Bipolar II Disorder, with clear episodes of hypomania and major depression that significantly impact her functioning. Her hypomanic symptoms are marked by increased energy, decreased need for sleep, and irritability, while her depressive episodes include low energy, hopelessness, and feelings of worthlessness.

- **Comorbid Anxiety Disorder**: Sarah's anxiety symptoms meet the DSM-5-TR criteria for an anxiety disorder due to their persistence, intensity, and impact on her life. Her anxiety includes general worry, panic episodes, and somatic symptoms (e.g., muscle tension, restlessness) that are unrelated to her mood fluctuations alone and often intensify during depressive phases.

Exclusion of Other Diagnoses:
- **Cyclothymic Disorder**: Sarah's clear episodes of hypomania and depression are more consistent with Bipolar II Disorder, ruling out cyclothymic disorder, which involves less intense, fluctuating mood symptoms.

- **Generalized Anxiety Disorder (GAD)** without Bipolar Disorder: Although Sarah has symptoms consistent with GAD, her mood instability and hypomanic/depressive episodes indicate that her anxiety is comorbid with Bipolar II Disorder rather than occurring independently.

- **Bipolar I Disorder**: Sarah has not experienced full manic episodes, differentiating her condition from Bipolar I Disorder.

Assessment Tools:
- **Mood Disorder Questionnaire (MDQ)**: This screening tool provided additional support for Sarah's history of mood episodes, confirming a consistent pattern of hypomanic and depressive phases over several years.
- **Hamilton Anxiety Rating Scale (HAM-A)**: This tool assessed the severity of Sarah's anxiety symptoms, revealing moderate to severe anxiety, including tension, panic, and worry, especially during depressive phases.

- **Structured Clinical Interview for DSM-5 Disorders (SCID-5)**: The SCID-5 was used to assess both mood and anxiety symptoms, verifying the presence of comorbid anxiety alongside Bipolar II Disorder.

Family Discussion: The clinician held a session with Sarah and her husband to discuss the diagnosis of Bipolar II Disorder with comorbid anxiety, explaining how the anxiety symptoms exacerbate her mood fluctuations. Treatment options, including mood stabilizers for bipolar symptoms and anxiolytics or specific forms of therapy for anxiety, were discussed. Sarah and her husband were educated on lifestyle modifications that could support symptom management, such as stress reduction techniques, routine-building, and mindfulness practices. Additionally, the clinician emphasized the importance of regular therapy for managing both mood and anxiety symptoms and for developing coping strategies.

Suggested Topics
- Overview of comorbidity in Bipolar Disorder and the effects of anxiety on mood regulation.
- Therapeutic approaches to managing bipolar disorder with comorbid anxiety, including CBT and pharmacotherapy.
- Lifestyle interventions and psychoeducation for improving anxiety and mood stability in bipolar disorder.

Chapter 16: Clinical Cases in Depressive Disorders

Introduction to Depressive Disorders

Depressive disorders encompass a range of mood disorders characterized primarily by persistent feelings of sadness, hopelessness, and a lack of interest or pleasure in daily activities. These conditions can significantly impair an individual's ability to function in personal, social, and professional spheres, affecting relationships, productivity, and overall quality of life. The DSM-5-TR classifies depressive disorders into several categories based on symptom duration, severity, and specific features, including major depressive disorder, persistent depressive disorder (dysthymia), and depression with psychotic features, among others.

The symptoms of depressive disorders vary widely, but common elements include changes in sleep, appetite, energy levels, concentration, and self-worth. Some forms of depression may involve additional unique features, such as psychotic symptoms or, in the case of postpartum depression, onset following childbirth. Depressive disorders are influenced by a combination of genetic, biochemical, environmental, and psychological factors, and they often occur alongside other mental health conditions, such as anxiety disorders or substance use disorders, which can complicate diagnosis and treatment.

Accurate diagnosis is essential, as depressive disorders respond to different treatment modalities, including psychotherapy, pharmacotherapy, and lifestyle changes. Specific subtypes, such as depression with psychotic features or postpartum depression, may require tailored approaches, integrating medical, psychological, and sometimes familial support. This chapter presents various clinical cases to illustrate the spectrum of depressive disorders, providing insights into diagnostic criteria, differential diagnoses, and effective treatment strategies. Through these cases, clinicians and students can deepen their understanding of the complex presentations of depression and explore evidence-based approaches to manage these impactful disorders effectively.

Case 16.1: Major Depressive Disorder

Patient Presentation
Patient: Emily, a 35-year-old female

Family Background: Emily lives alone and works as a high school English teacher. Known for her dedication to her students and love for literature, her friends and family have recently noticed a marked change in her mood and behavior. She has become increasingly isolated and unmotivated, and her family describes her as "a shadow of her former self." Emily has a history of mild depressive symptoms but has not previously sought treatment.

Key Symptoms:
- **Depressed Mood**: Emily reports feeling "overwhelmed by sadness" nearly every day for the past few months. She often cries and expresses a sense of hopelessness, describing her days as "emotionally exhausting."

- **Anhedonia**: She has lost interest in activities she once enjoyed, such as reading and spending time with her friends. Her disengagement is particularly noticeable in her teaching, where she struggles to maintain enthusiasm for her lessons.

- **Sleep Disturbances**: Emily reports difficulty falling asleep and frequent nighttime awakenings. She often wakes up feeling fatigued, despite getting several hours of sleep.

- **Changes in Appetite**: She has experienced a noticeable loss of appetite, leading to weight loss. She describes eating as a chore and says she "just doesn't feel hungry."

- **Low Energy and Fatigue**: Emily finds it increasingly difficult to get through her workday, often feeling exhausted after simple tasks.

- **Feelings of Worthlessness and Guilt**: She frequently blames herself for perceived failures, feeling inadequate in both her personal life and professional role.

Symptom Evolution:

Emily's symptoms began gradually six months ago, initially presenting as low energy and disinterest in social activities. Over time, her symptoms have intensified, affecting her ability to function at work and her interactions with family and friends. She initially attributed her feelings to work stress, but as her symptoms worsened, she began to feel that her sadness was pervasive and unmanageable.

Previous Interventions or Diagnoses:

Emily has never received formal mental health treatment, although she has occasionally experienced brief periods of low mood in the past, typically during stressful times. Her current depressive symptoms, however, are more severe and persistent than any prior experiences, prompting her family to encourage her to seek help.

Clinical Decision-Making Process

DSM-5-TR Diagnostic Criteria Considered:
- **Presence of Major Depressive Symptoms**: According to the DSM-5-TR, Major Depressive Disorder (MDD) is diagnosed when an individual experiences five or more symptoms (e.g., depressed mood, anhedonia, sleep disturbances, fatigue, and feelings of worthlessness) for at least two weeks. Emily meets these criteria, as she has experienced depressed mood, loss of interest, sleep problems, fatigue, appetite changes, and feelings of worthlessness nearly every day for over six months.

- **Significant Functional Impairment**: Emily's symptoms have affected her ability to perform her job effectively and have strained her social relationships, meeting the DSM-5-TR criterion of functional impairment.

Exclusion of Other Diagnoses:
- **Persistent Depressive Disorder (Dysthymia)**: Although Emily's symptoms have persisted for several months, the intensity and duration of her current depressive episode meet the threshold for MDD rather than the more chronic, less severe presentation of dysthymia.

- **Bipolar Disorder**: Emily has no history of manic or hypomanic episodes, ruling out bipolar disorder.

- **Adjustment Disorder with Depressed Mood**: Emily's symptoms are not clearly tied to a specific stressor, and the severity of her symptoms aligns more closely with MDD than with adjustment disorder.

Assessment Tools:
- **Beck Depression Inventory-II (BDI-II)**: This self-report tool assessed the severity of Emily's depressive symptoms. Her scores indicated severe depression, consistent with MDD.

- **Patient Health Questionnaire-9 (PHQ-9)**: The PHQ-9 provided additional insight into the frequency and impact of her depressive symptoms, further confirming the diagnosis of MDD.

- **Clinical Interview**: A structured interview was conducted to clarify Emily's symptom history and exclude other mental health conditions, confirming her presentation aligned with MDD.

Family Discussion: The clinician held a session with Emily and her family to explain Major Depressive Disorder, its symptoms, and the impact it has on daily functioning. The clinician discussed treatment options, including antidepressant therapy and cognitive-behavioral therapy (CBT), which could help Emily manage her symptoms. Emily's family was encouraged to provide a supportive environment and to check in on her progress, recognizing early signs of symptom recurrence. Psychoeducation on managing stress, maintaining a routine, and practicing self-care was also provided to help Emily stabilize her mood.

Suggested Topics
- Differentiating Major Depressive Disorder from Persistent Depressive Disorder.
- Overview of antidepressant options and considerations in MDD treatment.
- Cognitive-behavioral therapy techniques for managing Major Depressive Disorder.

Case 16.2: Persistent Depressive Disorder (Dysthymia)

Patient Presentation

Patient: Michael, a 42-year-old male

Family Background: Michael lives with his wife and two children. He works as an accountant and is described by his family as reserved and often "down." His wife notes that he rarely shows enthusiasm and has struggled with low mood for many years. He has few close friends and typically avoids social gatherings, preferring solitude.

Key Symptoms:

- **Chronic Low Mood**: Michael reports feeling "down" or "blue" most days for as long as he can remember, but especially in the last few years. He describes his mood as a "constant gray cloud," with only occasional brief moments of slight relief.

- **Low Self-Esteem**: He often feels inadequate and doubts his own abilities, especially at work. He worries excessively about making mistakes, even in routine tasks.

- **Fatigue and Low Energy**: Michael feels tired most of the time, struggling to find the energy to engage in family activities or even household tasks. He frequently describes feeling "drained."

- **Poor Appetite**: He has a reduced appetite, though he eats regularly due to his wife's encouragement. He has noticed slight weight loss but feels indifferent about it.

- **Hopelessness**: Michael expresses a sense of resignation about his mood, often telling his wife, "This is just how I am," and seeing little hope for improvement.

Symptom Evolution:

Michael's symptoms have been present for at least ten years, with periods of greater intensity interspersed with slightly improved moods. However, his mood has never been fully stable or "normal." Despite encouragement from his wife, he has resisted seeking help, attributing his mood to "stress" or his "personality." His symptoms have intensified over the past year, impacting his relationship with his children and causing increasing strain at work, prompting his wife to urge him to pursue an evaluation.

Previous Interventions or Diagnoses:

Michael has never received formal mental health treatment and has no prior diagnoses. His history of persistent low mood has been largely untreated, with his previous attempts to manage his symptoms on his own. His current condition is the first time he has seriously considered professional help.

Clinical Decision-Making Process

DSM-5-TR Diagnostic Criteria Considered:
- **Chronicity of Symptoms**: Persistent Depressive Disorder (Dysthymia) is diagnosed when depressive symptoms last for at least two years in adults, without a period of more than two consecutive months free from symptoms. Michael's prolonged low mood and associated symptoms clearly meet this duration requirement, as his symptoms have been consistently present for over a decade.

- **Depressive Symptoms**: Michael exhibits key symptoms of dysthymia, including low self-esteem, fatigue, poor appetite, low energy, and a pervasive sense of hopelessness. These symptoms meet the DSM-5-TR criteria for Persistent Depressive Disorder.

- **Functional Impairment**: His symptoms, while not as severe as those of Major Depressive Disorder, have a continuous negative impact on his work, social interactions, and family life, fulfilling the requirement of functional impairment associated with the disorder.

Exclusion of Other Diagnoses:
- **Major Depressive Disorder**: Although Michael's symptoms are persistent, they do not reach the intensity of Major Depressive Disorder. His low mood is more stable and chronic, without discrete, intense episodes.

- **Cyclothymic Disorder**: Cyclothymic disorder was ruled out due to the lack of hypomanic symptoms. Michael's mood remains consistently low without fluctuating to any elevated state.

- **Adjustment Disorder with Depressed Mood**: Adjustment Disorder was ruled out as Michael's symptoms are not tied to a specific recent life stressor and have been consistently present over many years.

Assessment Tools:
- **Patient Health Questionnaire-9 (PHQ-9)**: The PHQ-9 was used to assess the severity of Michael's depressive symptoms. His scores were consistent with mild to moderate chronic depression, in line with Persistent Depressive Disorder.

- **Beck Depression Inventory-II (BDI-II)**: This inventory confirmed the presence of chronic low-grade depressive symptoms, supporting the diagnosis of dysthymia.
- **Structured Clinical Interview for DSM-5 Disorders (SCID-5)**: The SCID-5 was used to evaluate Michael's mood history and verify the duration and consistency of symptoms. It confirmed that his symptoms met the criteria for Persistent Depressive Disorder.

Family Discussion: The clinician held a session with Michael and his wife to discuss Persistent Depressive Disorder, explaining the chronic nature of the condition and its treatment options. Treatment strategies, including antidepressants and cognitive-behavioral therapy (CBT), were discussed as means to help Michael gradually improve his mood stability and quality of life. The clinician provided guidance on setting realistic goals and managing expectations, given the chronic nature of his symptoms, and encouraged Michael to maintain open communication with his family to aid in his treatment journey.

Suggested Topics
- Understanding the differences between Persistent Depressive Disorder and Major Depressive Disorder.
- Overview of therapeutic approaches for managing dysthymia, including CBT and antidepressant treatment.
- Family support and psychoeducation in Persistent Depressive Disorder management.

Case 16.3: Depression with Psychotic Features

Patient Presentation

Patient: Linda, a 50-year-old female

Family Background: Linda lives with her husband and has two adult children who live nearby. She works part-time as an administrative assistant and has always been regarded as responsible and diligent. Recently, however, her family and coworkers have noticed significant changes in her mood and behavior. Her family describes her as becoming increasingly withdrawn, anxious, and suspicious over the past few months.

Key Symptoms:
- **Severe Depressive Symptoms**: Linda exhibits symptoms of severe depression, including pervasive sadness, lack of energy, anhedonia, and frequent crying spells. She expresses feelings of worthlessness and hopelessness, believing that her life has lost all meaning.

- **Psychotic Features**: Linda reports experiencing auditory hallucinations, specifically hearing voices that criticize her and reinforce her feelings of inadequacy. She has also developed a delusional belief that she is being punished for her "failures" as a mother and wife. These beliefs and hallucinations worsen when she is alone or in quiet settings.

- **Cognitive Impairment**: Linda has difficulty concentrating and often forgets routine tasks, such as paying bills or following up on her work responsibilities. Her cognitive difficulties have become apparent to her family and coworkers, who have noticed her making mistakes and struggling to keep up with her usual tasks.

Symptom Evolution:

Linda's symptoms emerged approximately three months ago, beginning with low energy and a noticeable decrease in motivation. Over time, her mood deteriorated further, and she started expressing feelings of guilt and hopelessness. In the past month, she began hearing voices and developed persistent beliefs that she was a failure, believing that these experiences were "proof" of her unworthiness. Her family became increasingly concerned when Linda shared her belief that she deserved to be punished and that her suffering was a form of retribution.

Previous Interventions or Diagnoses:

Linda has a history of mild depression, for which she received brief counseling in her early thirties. However, she has no history of severe depressive episodes, psychosis, or any other psychiatric condition. Her current symptoms represent her first experience with psychotic features.

Clinical Decision-Making Process

DSM-5-TR Diagnostic Criteria Considered:
- **Major Depressive Episode with Psychotic Features**: According to the DSM-5-TR, Major Depressive Disorder with Psychotic Features is diagnosed when an individual meets the criteria for a major depressive episode and experiences delusions or hallucinations. Linda exhibits symptoms of a severe depressive episode and psychotic features, such as auditory hallucinations and delusional guilt, consistent with this diagnosis.

- **Mood-Congruent Psychotic Features**: Linda's delusions and hallucinations are congruent with her depressive mood, reinforcing her feelings of worthlessness and guilt. This congruence is characteristic of Major Depressive Disorder with mood-congruent psychotic features.

Exclusion of Other Diagnoses:
- **Schizoaffective Disorder**: Schizoaffective Disorder was ruled out because Linda's psychotic symptoms occur exclusively during her depressive episode. In schizoaffective disorder, psychotic symptoms must occur independently of mood episodes.

- **Bipolar Disorder with Psychotic Features**: Linda has no history of mania or hypomania, excluding a diagnosis of Bipolar Disorder with psychotic features.

- **Psychotic Disorder due to a Medical Condition**: A thorough medical examination, including lab tests and neuroimaging, ruled out any underlying medical or neurological conditions that could account for her psychotic symptoms.

Assessment Tools:
- **Hamilton Depression Rating Scale (HDRS)**: This scale was used to assess the severity of Linda's depressive symptoms. Her high scores confirmed the presence of severe depression, supporting the diagnosis of Major Depressive Disorder with psychotic features.

- **Brief Psychiatric Rating Scale (BPRS)**: The BPRS helped evaluate the severity of Linda's psychotic symptoms, including auditory hallucinations and delusional beliefs, further corroborating the diagnosis.

- **Structured Clinical Interview for DSM-5 Disorders (SCID-5)**: The SCID-5 was utilized to confirm the criteria for Major Depressive Disorder with psychotic features and exclude other psychotic and mood disorders.

Family Discussion: The clinician met with Linda and her family to discuss the diagnosis and provide insight into her experiences of depression with psychotic features. Treatment options, including a combination of antidepressants and antipsychotic medications, were discussed, emphasizing the importance of addressing both her mood and psychotic symptoms. Linda's family was provided with education on recognizing warning signs and encouraged to support her through regular follow-ups and therapy. Psychoeducation also covered the need for routine and stress management to aid in her recovery process.

Suggested Topics
- Understanding mood-congruent vs. mood-incongruent psychotic features in depressive disorders.
- Pharmacological treatments for Major Depressive Disorder with psychotic features, including antidepressants and antipsychotics.
- Role of family support and psychoeducation in managing psychotic features within depressive episodes.

Case 16.4: Postpartum Depression

Patient Presentation
Patient: Rachel, a 30-year-old female

Family Background: Rachel recently gave birth to her first child two months ago and lives with her husband in a supportive household. Although Rachel and her husband were excited about becoming parents, she has struggled to adjust to motherhood and has begun feeling overwhelmed and disconnected. Her husband, who has taken some time off work to support her, has grown concerned as Rachel's mood has worsened since the birth of their baby.

Key Symptoms:
- **Persistent Sadness and Tearfulness**: Rachel reports feeling sad and tearful almost every day. She often cries without a specific reason and describes feeling an overwhelming sense of sadness that she cannot explain.
- **Loss of Interest and Anhedonia**: She has lost interest in activities she previously enjoyed, including her hobbies and socializing. She also feels detached from her baby, struggling to bond and feeling little joy in caring for her child.
- **Fatigue and Sleep Disturbances**: Although Rachel's baby sleeps relatively well, she finds it difficult to sleep even when the baby is resting, often lying awake with worries and negative thoughts. She experiences fatigue throughout the day, which worsens her mood.
- **Feelings of Inadequacy and Guilt**: Rachel frequently expresses feelings of guilt, believing she is a "bad mother" for struggling to connect with her baby and doubting her abilities as a parent.
- **Irritability and Anxiety**: Rachel feels irritable and anxious, particularly around feeding and taking care of the baby. She worries constantly about her parenting skills and feels on edge, as if she is failing her child.

Symptom Evolution:

Rachel's symptoms began within a few weeks after delivery. Initially, she experienced "baby blues," feeling somewhat emotional and tired, which she believed was normal. However, her mood did not improve, and within a month, her sadness and anxiety intensified, affecting her ability to care for herself and her baby. Her husband noticed that she rarely smiled, even when interacting with the baby, and seemed increasingly withdrawn.

Previous Interventions or Diagnoses:

Rachel has no previous history of mental health issues, and her pregnancy was generally healthy with no complications. This current episode marks her first experience with a depressive condition. Due to her worsening mood, her husband encouraged her to seek help.

Clinical Decision-Making Process

DSM-5-TR Diagnostic Criteria Considered:
- **Major Depressive Episode with Postpartum Onset**: According to the DSM-5-TR, postpartum depression is considered a subtype of Major Depressive Disorder, specified by its onset within four weeks of childbirth. Rachel's symptoms of sadness, guilt, fatigue, and anhedonia align with a major depressive episode that began within the postpartum period.

- **Functional Impairment**: Rachel's depressive symptoms significantly impact her ability to care for her child, maintain a routine, and engage in social or family activities, fulfilling the DSM-5-TR criterion for functional impairment.

Exclusion of Other Diagnoses:
- **Baby Blues**: Although "baby blues" are common after childbirth, they typically resolve within two weeks. Rachel's symptoms persisted and intensified beyond this period, differentiating her condition from the transient emotional changes associated with "baby blues."
- **Persistent Depressive Disorder (Dysthymia)**: Rachel's symptoms are specific to the postpartum period and have not been present for the extended duration required for a diagnosis of Persistent Depressive Disorder.

- **Adjustment Disorder with Depressed Mood**: Rachel's symptoms meet the criteria for a major depressive episode rather than an adjustment disorder, given the severity, duration, and impact on her functioning.

Assessment Tools:
- **Edinburgh Postnatal Depression Scale (EPDS)**: This self-report tool, specifically designed for postpartum depression, was administered to evaluate the severity of Rachel's depressive symptoms. Her high score indicated significant postpartum depression, supporting the diagnosis.

- **Patient Health Questionnaire-9 (PHQ-9)**: The PHQ-9 was used to assess the severity and frequency of her depressive symptoms, further confirming a major depressive episode.

- **Clinical Interview**: Through a structured interview, Rachel's symptom history and functional impairment were clarified, confirming the diagnosis of Major Depressive Disorder with postpartum onset.

Family Discussion: The clinician met with Rachel and her husband to discuss postpartum depression, its causes, and treatment options. The clinician provided reassurance that postpartum depression is treatable and not a reflection of Rachel's abilities as a mother. Treatment options, including antidepressants (safe for breastfeeding) and cognitive-behavioral therapy (CBT), were discussed. The clinician also recommended family support and counseling to help Rachel feel more supported and confident in her new role. Her husband was advised on ways to provide additional support and encouraged to monitor Rachel's symptoms for any worsening or emergent signs.

Suggested Topics
- Overview of postpartum depression and its differentiation from "baby blues."
- Pharmacological and therapeutic approaches for treating postpartum depression, including breastfeeding-safe antidepressants.
- The role of family support and psychoeducation in the management and recovery of postpartum depression.

Case 16.5: Substance-Induced Depressive Disorder

Patient Presentation
Patient: James, a 48-year-old male

Family Background: James is divorced and lives alone, working as a construction foreman. Known for his strong work ethic and resilience, he has recently shown signs of mood instability, withdrawal, and increased irritability. His sister, who lives nearby, has become concerned about his behavior, especially given recent life changes and his history of heavy alcohol consumption.

Key Symptoms:
- **Persistent Low Mood**: James reports feeling persistently "down" and unmotivated. He describes his mood as "numb" and expresses little interest in daily activities, which has negatively impacted his work performance and social life.

- **Anhedonia**: He finds little pleasure in activities he once enjoyed, such as fishing and spending time with friends, preferring instead to be alone and disengaged.

- **Sleep Disruption**: James experiences frequent insomnia and has difficulty maintaining a regular sleep schedule. He reports waking up multiple times during the night and feeling unrefreshed in the morning.

- **Fatigue and Low Energy**: James feels physically drained throughout the day, lacking the energy to complete even simple tasks.

- **Feelings of Guilt and Hopelessness**: He expresses regret over his past choices, particularly his alcohol use, and worries that he is "too far gone" to improve his situation. These feelings contribute to a pervasive sense of hopelessness.

Symptom Evolution:

James's depressive symptoms began worsening approximately three months ago, shortly after a period of increased alcohol consumption following a difficult breakup. Although he has had periods of mild low mood in the past, this is the first time his symptoms have persisted and intensified over an extended period. His sister notes that his alcohol intake has increased steadily over the past six months, especially in the evenings after work, with drinking becoming a nightly routine.

Previous Interventions or Diagnoses:

James has no formal history of depressive disorders or mental health treatment. However, he has a long-standing history of heavy alcohol use, which has occasionally led to conflicts at work and strained relationships. He has never sought treatment for his drinking habits, often downplaying their impact on his life.

Clinical Decision-Making Process

DSM-5-TR Diagnostic Criteria Considered:
- **Substance-Induced Depressive Disorder**: According to the DSM-5-TR, a diagnosis of Substance-Induced Depressive Disorder can be made when depressive symptoms develop during or shortly after substance use and persist beyond the expected duration of intoxication or withdrawal. In James's case, his depressive symptoms align with his pattern of increased alcohol use, suggesting that his low mood, anhedonia, and hopelessness are directly linked to his substance use.

- **Temporal Association with Substance Use**: James's symptoms worsened in parallel with his increased alcohol consumption, particularly during the past three months. This temporal relationship supports a diagnosis of Substance-Induced Depressive Disorder.

- **Functional Impairment**: James's symptoms interfere with his daily functioning, affecting his work, social relationships, and overall quality of life, fulfilling the DSM-5-TR criterion for significant functional impairment.

Exclusion of Other Diagnoses:
- **Major Depressive Disorder (MDD)**: Although James exhibits symptoms of depression, his symptoms appear closely tied to his alcohol use. MDD was ruled out as his mood symptoms are likely induced by his substance use rather than being primary.

- **Persistent Depressive Disorder (Dysthymia)**: James's symptoms emerged relatively recently and are closely linked to his alcohol use, differentiating his case from the chronic, long-term low mood seen in dysthymia.

- **Adjustment Disorder with Depressed Mood**: Although his recent breakup likely contributed to increased drinking, James's symptoms align more with a substance-induced mood disorder rather than a direct response to a life stressor.

Assessment Tools:

- **Alcohol Use Disorders Identification Test (AUDIT)**: The AUDIT was used to assess James's alcohol consumption patterns, confirming heavy use that has contributed to his current mood state.

- **Patient Health Questionnaire-9 (PHQ-9)**: This tool assessed the severity of his depressive symptoms. His scores indicated moderate to severe depression, further supporting the diagnosis of a substance-induced mood disorder.

- **Clinical Interview**: Through a structured interview, James's mood symptoms, alcohol use history, and functional impairment were clarified. The interview confirmed the link between his depressive symptoms and increased alcohol use.

Family Discussion: The clinician held a session with James and his sister to discuss the diagnosis and explain how alcohol can exacerbate or induce depressive symptoms. Treatment options were discussed, with an emphasis on the importance of reducing or eliminating alcohol use to improve his mood. The clinician recommended a dual approach, addressing both substance use and mood symptoms, with possible treatment options including motivational interviewing, cognitive-behavioral therapy (CBT), and support groups. His sister was encouraged to support James by fostering a non-judgmental environment and helping him access resources for managing his substance use.

Suggested Topics
- Understanding the relationship between substance use and mood disorders.
- Treatment approaches for Substance-Induced Depressive Disorder, including behavioral therapies and support groups.
- The impact of alcohol on mood regulation and strategies for managing alcohol-related mood changes.

Chapter 17: **Clinical Cases in Anxiety Disorders**

Introduction to Anxiety Disorders

Anxiety disorders encompass a range of mental health conditions characterized by excessive fear, worry, or avoidance that interferes with daily functioning. While occasional anxiety is a natural response to stress, anxiety disorders involve persistent and often disproportionate responses to perceived threats or stressors. These disorders can lead to significant distress and functional impairment, affecting an individual's ability to work, socialize, and maintain relationships.

The DSM-5-TR categorizes anxiety disorders into several specific types, including Generalized Anxiety Disorder (GAD), characterized by pervasive and chronic worry; Panic Disorder, marked by recurrent panic attacks and intense fear of future attacks; Social Anxiety Disorder, involving fear of social situations; Agoraphobia, where individuals avoid situations they believe may be difficult to escape; and Separation Anxiety Disorder, often seen in children but can persist into adulthood, involving distress when separated from loved ones. Each subtype has unique symptoms, yet all share a core component of irrational fear or avoidance.

Anxiety disorders are often comorbid with other mental health conditions, including mood disorders, substance use disorders, and other anxiety disorders, which can complicate diagnosis and treatment. Identifying and treating anxiety disorders requires a comprehensive approach, as they may also manifest with somatic symptoms such as muscle tension, headaches, and gastrointestinal issues, which can lead to misdiagnosis or underdiagnosis.

This chapter presents clinical cases illustrating various anxiety disorders, detailing their presentation, diagnostic process, and treatment strategies. By exploring these cases, clinicians and students can gain a deeper understanding of how anxiety disorders manifest in real-life settings and learn about evidence-based approaches for effective management.

Case 17.1: Generalized Anxiety Disorder

Patient Presentation

Patient: Laura, a 32-year-old female

Family Background: Laura lives with her husband and 5-year-old son in an urban area. She works as a marketing manager and is known for her meticulousness and attention to detail. Recently, her husband and coworkers have noticed that she seems increasingly anxious and withdrawn, with frequent expressions of worry about various aspects of her life. Laura describes herself as a "chronic worrier" and feels overwhelmed by constant feelings of dread.

Key Symptoms:

- **Excessive Worry**: Laura reports feeling anxious about numerous aspects of her life, including her job, finances, family health, and her child's future. Her worries are often out of proportion to the actual situation, and she finds it challenging to control or stop these thoughts.

- **Physical Symptoms**: She experiences frequent muscle tension, headaches, and gastrointestinal discomfort, which she attributes to her anxiety. These symptoms often worsen during particularly stressful periods at work or at home.

- **Sleep Difficulties**: Laura has trouble falling asleep due to racing thoughts and frequently wakes up in the night, feeling restless and tired in the morning.

- **Irritability and Fatigue**: The constant worrying has left Laura feeling exhausted and irritable, especially in the evenings. She has difficulty focusing on her tasks at work and finds herself double-checking her work excessively to avoid making mistakes.

Symptom Evolution:

Laura's symptoms have been present for as long as she can remember, but they became more pronounced following the birth of her son. Over the past year, her worries have intensified, leading her to constantly monitor her family's well-being and double-check tasks at work. She initially attributed these feelings to general life stress but has recently realized that her anxiety is affecting her health and relationships.

Previous Interventions or Diagnoses:

Laura has never received formal treatment for her anxiety. She did attempt self-help techniques, such as mindfulness exercises, which provided temporary relief but did not address the underlying worry. Her increased irritability and fatigue eventually led her to seek a professional evaluation.

Clinical Decision-Making Process

DSM-5-TR Diagnostic Criteria Considered:
- **Excessive Worry and Anxiety**: According to the DSM-5-TR, Generalized Anxiety Disorder (GAD) is characterized by excessive worry about a variety of topics, lasting for at least six months and occurring more days than not. Laura meets these criteria, as her anxiety is pervasive, difficult to control, and has persisted for over a year.

- **Associated Symptoms**: Laura's additional symptoms—muscle tension, fatigue, irritability, and sleep disturbance—are consistent with the diagnostic criteria for GAD, which requires at least three of these associated symptoms in adults.

- **Functional Impairment**: Laura's anxiety significantly interferes with her work performance, sleep, and relationships, meeting the DSM-5-TR criterion for functional impairment.

Exclusion of Other Diagnoses:
- **Panic Disorder**: While Laura experiences physical symptoms of anxiety, they are chronic rather than episodic and are not associated with sudden panic attacks, ruling out Panic Disorder.

- **Obsessive-Compulsive Disorder (OCD)**: Laura's repetitive behaviors, such as double-checking, stem from anxiety about making mistakes rather than specific, intrusive obsessions. Her symptoms align more closely with generalized anxiety than OCD.

- **Adjustment Disorder with Anxiety**: While Laura's anxiety worsened following life changes, such as the birth of her son, her pervasive and long-standing worry suggests a diagnosis of GAD rather than an adjustment disorder.

Assessment Tools:
- **Generalized Anxiety Disorder-7 (GAD-7)**: This screening tool assessed the severity of Laura's anxiety, confirming high levels consistent with GAD.

- **Beck Anxiety Inventory (BAI)**: The BAI provided additional insight into the physical symptoms of Laura's anxiety, supporting the diagnosis.

- **Structured Clinical Interview for DSM-5 Disorders (SCID-5)**: The SCID-5 was used to confirm that Laura's symptoms met the criteria for GAD, and it helped rule out other potential anxiety disorders.

Family Discussion: The clinician discussed the diagnosis with Laura and her husband, emphasizing the chronic nature of GAD and the need for comprehensive treatment. Options were discussed, including cognitive-behavioral therapy (CBT), which could help Laura manage her worry patterns, and possibly medication to address her symptoms. The clinician provided Laura's husband with guidance on how to support her, encouraging open communication and involvement in her therapeutic journey. Psychoeducation covered relaxation techniques and self-care practices to help Laura reduce the physical impact of her anxiety.

Suggested Topics
- The cognitive-behavioral approach to treating Generalized Anxiety Disorder.
- Understanding the role of physical symptoms in GAD and their management.
- Differentiating Generalized Anxiety Disorder from other anxiety disorders and adjustment disorders.

Case 17.2: Panic Disorder

Patient Presentation
Patient: Mark, a 27-year-old male

Family Background: Mark is single and lives alone in a small city apartment. He works as a junior accountant, a job he typically enjoys. Mark has always been generally calm and focused, but recently, he has started experiencing sudden, intense episodes of fear and physical symptoms that have left him feeling anxious about his well-being. His parents, who live nearby, are worried about his health and have encouraged him to seek help.

Key Symptoms:
- **Recurrent Panic Attacks**: Mark reports experiencing sudden episodes of intense fear, which seem to come out of nowhere. During these attacks, he feels as though he's "losing control" and even worries that he might be having a heart attack. His attacks are characterized by a rapid heartbeat, sweating, shortness of breath, and a feeling of impending doom.

- **Fear of Future Attacks**: The fear of experiencing another panic attack has caused Mark to avoid certain situations, such as crowded places or enclosed spaces like elevators, which he associates with his attacks. He describes feeling on edge, constantly worried that an attack might happen again.

- **Physical Symptoms**: During an attack, Mark experiences chest pain, dizziness, and feelings of detachment from reality. These symptoms are severe enough to leave him exhausted and anxious for hours afterward.

Symptom Evolution:

Mark's first panic attack occurred around six months ago while he was at a busy subway station. Since then, he has had frequent attacks, with no clear pattern as to when they will occur. Initially, he brushed them off as isolated incidents, but as the attacks increased in frequency, he began worrying more about when the next one might happen. His fear of having another attack has led him to avoid places where he has had attacks before, such as subways and crowded stores, causing noticeable changes in his lifestyle.

Previous Interventions or Diagnoses:

Mark has no previous mental health diagnoses and has never sought psychiatric treatment. He did visit his primary care doctor after his first attack, where cardiac and other medical issues were ruled out, leading his doctor to suggest that his symptoms might be related to anxiety.

Clinical Decision-Making Process

DSM-5-TR Diagnostic Criteria Considered:
- **Panic Attacks**: According to the DSM-5-TR, Panic Disorder is characterized by recurrent, unexpected panic attacks. Mark's experiences meet this criterion, as he has frequent episodes of intense fear and physical symptoms that seem to occur without a clear trigger.

- **Persistent Concern about Additional Attacks**: Mark's ongoing worry about future attacks and his behavioral changes, such as avoiding crowded places, support the DSM-5-TR criteria for Panic Disorder. His concern about having additional attacks significantly impacts his daily life, further supporting the diagnosis.

- **Functional Impairment**: Mark's avoidance behaviors and his constant worry about potential panic attacks interfere with his ability to go about his daily routine, fulfilling the DSM-5-TR criterion for functional impairment.

Exclusion of Other Diagnoses:
- **Agoraphobia**: Although Mark avoids certain places due to fear of having a panic attack, his avoidance is tied specifically to his panic symptoms rather than a broader fear of being unable to escape or find help. His symptoms align more closely with Panic Disorder than with agoraphobia.

- **Generalized Anxiety Disorder (GAD)**: While Mark experiences anxiety, it is specific to panic attacks rather than generalized worry about multiple life areas, ruling out GAD.

- **Specific Phobia**: Mark's fear is not tied to a specific object or situation but is instead centered around his fear of experiencing another panic attack, differentiating it from specific phobias.

Assessment Tools:
- **Panic Disorder Severity Scale (PDSS)**: This scale helped assess the frequency, severity, and functional impact of Mark's panic attacks, confirming a level consistent with Panic Disorder.

- **Beck Anxiety Inventory (BAI)**: The BAI provided additional information on the severity of his anxiety symptoms during and between attacks, supporting the diagnosis.

- **Clinical Interview**: A structured clinical interview was conducted to clarify Mark's panic symptoms, history, and functional impairment, confirming that his experiences align with the DSM-5-TR criteria for Panic Disorder.

Family Discussion: The clinician met with Mark and his parents to discuss the diagnosis of Panic Disorder and its impact on his life. Treatment options, including cognitive-behavioral therapy (CBT) with a focus on exposure therapy, were discussed to help Mark confront and reduce his fear of future attacks. The clinician explained the cycle of panic attacks and how avoidance can reinforce his anxiety, and Mark's parents were encouraged to provide support without enabling his avoidance behaviors. The clinician also discussed relaxation techniques and grounding exercises as tools for managing symptoms during an attack.

Suggested Topics
- Cognitive-behavioral therapy techniques, particularly exposure therapy, for managing Panic Disorder.
- Understanding the physiological and psychological components of panic attacks.
- Role of family support and strategies to prevent reinforcement of avoidance behaviors in individuals with Panic Disorder.

Case 17.3: Social Anxiety Disorder

Patient Presentation

Patient: Anna, a 24-year-old female

Family Background: Anna recently moved out of her parents' home to a small apartment in the city. She works as a graphic designer and is recognized for her creativity, although she is reserved and prefers working on tasks independently. Over the past few years, Anna's family and friends have noticed her tendency to avoid social situations and gatherings, even with people she knows well. Anna describes herself as "extremely self-conscious" and feels intense fear in situations where she believes she will be judged.

Key Symptoms:

- **Fear of Social Situations**: Anna experiences overwhelming fear in social and performance situations, including work meetings, social gatherings, and public speaking. She worries excessively about embarrassing herself or being perceived as inadequate, and her fear is often disproportionate to the situation.

- **Physical Symptoms of Anxiety**: In social settings, Anna experiences physical symptoms such as sweating, trembling, nausea, and a racing heart. She describes feeling "paralyzed" by her anxiety, especially when she believes others are watching her.

- **Avoidance Behaviors**: Anna often avoids social situations, including casual socializing with colleagues or going to events where she might need to interact with people. She turns down invitations and has missed opportunities for advancement at work due to her fear of presenting in meetings.

- **Low Self-Esteem and Self-Criticism**: Anna constantly worries that others view her negatively and frequently criticizes her own social performance. After an interaction, she ruminates over her perceived mistakes, reinforcing her belief that she's socially inadequate.

Symptom Evolution:

Anna's social anxiety began in high school and has progressively worsened over time. She initially struggled only with public speaking but now finds nearly all social interactions anxiety-provoking. Her avoidance behaviors have increased since starting her job, where she has missed important networking events and presentation opportunities. This avoidance has impacted her personal life as well, as she has few close friends and rarely participates in social activities outside of work.

Previous Interventions or Diagnoses:

Anna has no prior history of psychiatric treatment, although she has been aware of her social anxiety for several years. Recently, her job performance has begun to suffer, and her supervisor suggested that she seek help to manage her anxiety.

Clinical Decision-Making Process

DSM-5-TR Diagnostic Criteria Considered:
- **Marked Fear of Social Situations**: According to the DSM-5-TR, Social Anxiety Disorder is diagnosed when there is a marked and persistent fear of social situations in which the individual feels exposed to possible scrutiny by others. Anna's fear of being judged or embarrassed in a variety of social settings meets this criterion.

- **Avoidance and Distress in Social Situations**: Anna avoids many social situations due to her anxiety, which interferes with her career and personal life, meeting the criterion for avoidance and functional impairment.

- **Duration and Impact**: Anna's anxiety has persisted for several years, affecting her life in significant ways, including her professional growth and social relationships. This chronic impact fulfills the DSM-5-TR requirement for Social Anxiety Disorder.

Exclusion of Other Diagnoses:
- **Generalized Anxiety Disorder (GAD)**: Although Anna experiences anxiety, it is specifically related to social situations and does not include general, pervasive worry across multiple areas of her life, differentiating it from GAD.

- **Panic Disorder**: While Anna experiences physical symptoms of anxiety in social settings, she does not experience unexpected, recurring panic attacks, ruling out Panic Disorder.

- **Avoidant Personality Disorder**: Anna's avoidance is specific to social and performance situations rather than pervasive avoidance across all interactions, and she does not exhibit other core characteristics of Avoidant Personality Disorder.

Assessment Tools:
- **Social Phobia Inventory (SPIN)**: This tool assessed the severity of Anna's social anxiety symptoms, confirming a high level of anxiety specifically related to social situations.

- **Liebowitz Social Anxiety Scale (LSAS)**: The LSAS helped evaluate Anna's degree of fear and avoidance across different social situations, further supporting the diagnosis of Social Anxiety Disorder.

- **Clinical Interview**: Through a structured clinical interview, Anna's social anxiety symptoms, avoidance behaviors, and associated self-criticism were clarified, confirming that her experiences align with DSM-5-TR criteria for Social Anxiety Disorder.

Family Discussion: Anna's clinician met with her to discuss her diagnosis of Social Anxiety Disorder, exploring the factors contributing to her condition and treatment options. Cognitive-behavioral therapy (CBT) with a focus on exposure therapy was recommended to help Anna confront her fear of social situations gradually. The clinician also discussed self-compassion techniques to address her self-critical thoughts after social interactions. Psychoeducation was provided to help Anna understand the nature of social anxiety, and she was encouraged to gradually engage in social settings with supportive friends or family members.

Suggested Topics
- Cognitive-behavioral therapy (CBT) techniques for Social Anxiety Disorder, with an emphasis on exposure therapy.
- Differentiating Social Anxiety Disorder from Generalized Anxiety Disorder and Avoidant Personality Disorder.
- Self-compassion and strategies for reducing self-criticism in Social Anxiety Disorder.

Case 17.4: Agoraphobia

Patient Presentation

Patient: John, a 38-year-old male

Family Background: John lives with his wife and two children in a suburban area. Once an active and social person, John has recently become increasingly reluctant to leave his home. He works remotely as a software developer and has structured his daily routine to avoid going out. His wife has grown concerned as he now refuses to accompany the family to routine activities like grocery shopping or family outings.

Key Symptoms:

- **Intense Fear of Being in Situations Where Escape Might Be Difficult**: John feels extreme anxiety at the thought of leaving his home, particularly when imagining places like crowded stores, theaters, or public transportation. He fears he would be unable to escape or find help if he were to experience panic symptoms.

- **Avoidance of Public Places**: Over the past few months, John has avoided visiting most public places. He declines invitations from friends and reschedules medical appointments unless absolutely necessary. Even driving his car has become a challenge, as he worries about being trapped in traffic without a way to quickly leave.

- **Physical Symptoms of Anxiety**: When in a situation that feels unsafe or where escape might be difficult, John experiences a racing heart, dizziness, nausea, and intense feelings of dread. These physical symptoms further reinforce his fear of leaving home.

Symptom Evolution:

John's symptoms began around a year ago following a severe panic attack he experienced while in a crowded mall. Initially, he simply avoided malls, but over time, his anxiety expanded to other locations. Now, his fear is generalized to almost any place outside his home, and he experiences anxiety at the thought of leaving his familiar environment. His avoidance behaviors have steadily increased, causing significant strain on his family and limiting his social and daily functioning.

Previous Interventions or Diagnoses:

John has no history of psychiatric treatment prior to his current symptoms. After experiencing his initial panic attack, he attempted to manage his anxiety independently, but his avoidance behaviors have gradually intensified. His family has encouraged him to seek professional help, recognizing the impact his anxiety is having on his life and relationships.

Clinical Decision-Making Process

DSM-5-TR Diagnostic Criteria Considered:
- **Marked Fear or Anxiety about Situations Where Escape Might Be Difficult**: According to the DSM-5-TR, Agoraphobia is characterized by intense fear or anxiety about two or more situations such as using public transportation, being in open or enclosed spaces, standing in line, or being in a crowd. John's fear of being in these situations, especially those that involve crowds or closed spaces, meets this criterion.

- **Avoidance of Feared Situations**: John's avoidance of public places, travel, and even everyday tasks like grocery shopping is significant. His avoidance impacts his ability to function normally and restricts his movement outside the home, meeting the DSM-5-TR criterion for agoraphobic avoidance.

- **Functional Impairment**: John's anxiety and avoidance behavior significantly limit his lifestyle, preventing him from participating in family activities, social events, and routine errands. This functional impairment aligns with the DSM-5-TR criteria for agoraphobia.

Exclusion of Other Diagnoses:
- **Panic Disorder**: Although John initially experienced a panic attack in a public place, his current fear centers around situations where he feels escape might be difficult, regardless of whether a panic attack occurs. Panic Disorder was ruled out as his anxiety is now primarily related to avoidance rather than repeated panic attacks.

- **Social Anxiety Disorder**: John's avoidance is not motivated by fear of social scrutiny or judgment but rather by fear of being trapped or unable to escape. This distinction helps differentiate his symptoms from Social Anxiety Disorder.

- **Specific Phobia**: While his anxiety is specific to certain situations, the broad range of environments he avoids aligns more closely with Agoraphobia than with Specific Phobia, which typically involves a more limited set of specific triggers.

Assessment Tools:
- **Agoraphobia Scale (AS)**: This tool assessed John's levels of fear and avoidance related to various agoraphobic situations, confirming a high degree of anxiety in situations where escape might be challenging.

- **Panic Disorder Severity Scale (PDSS)**: Although originally developed for Panic Disorder, the PDSS provided insight into John's experiences of panic symptoms and situational avoidance, supporting the diagnosis of Agoraphobia without recurring panic attacks.

- **Clinical Interview**: A structured interview was conducted to clarify John's avoidance behaviors, physical symptoms, and history of panic experiences, confirming that his symptoms align with DSM-5-TR criteria for Agoraphobia.

Family Discussion: The clinician met with John and his wife to discuss Agoraphobia, its symptoms, and the effects on his daily life. Treatment options, including cognitive-behavioral therapy (CBT) with exposure therapy, were discussed to gradually help John confront his fear of public spaces. The clinician explained how avoidance reinforces anxiety and worked with John and his family to develop a gradual plan to approach feared situations. His wife was encouraged to provide support and understanding as John begins exposure-based treatment and learns to manage his symptoms outside the home.

Suggested Topics
- Cognitive-behavioral therapy (CBT) techniques for Agoraphobia, focusing on exposure therapy.
- Understanding the cycle of avoidance and reinforcement in Agoraphobia.
- Differentiating Agoraphobia from Panic Disorder and Social Anxiety Disorder.

Case 17.5: Separation Anxiety Disorder

Patient Presentation

Patient: Mia, an 11-year-old female

Family Background: Mia lives with her parents and younger brother. She has always been close to her family, particularly her mother, with whom she has a very strong bond. Over the past year, her parents have noticed that Mia has become increasingly anxious and distressed when separated from her mother, even in familiar settings such as school or with family friends. Her mother reports that Mia often cries and clings to her whenever she has to leave, expressing fears about their safety and well-being.

Key Symptoms:

- **Excessive Distress upon Separation**: Mia experiences intense emotional distress whenever she anticipates being separated from her mother. This distress includes crying, clinginess, and repeated reassurances about her mother's safety.

- **Persistent Worry about Harm to Loved Ones**: Mia expresses ongoing fears that something bad will happen to her mother or other family members when she is away from them. She often imagines accidents or dangers, which exacerbate her anxiety.

- **Physical Symptoms of Anxiety**: When Mia is separated from her mother, she experiences stomachaches, headaches, and nausea, which sometimes lead her to ask to go home early from school.

- **Difficulty Sleeping Alone**: Mia struggles to sleep in her own bed and often requests to sleep in her parents' room. On the rare occasions that she sleeps in her own room, she frequently gets up to check on her parents or seeks reassurance from them.

Symptom Evolution:

Mia's symptoms began to intensify after her grandmother passed away unexpectedly. Since then, she has become increasingly fearful about losing her mother or family members. Initially, her symptoms were limited to occasional worries, but over time, they became more pervasive. Her anxiety now affects her ability to attend school consistently, complete assignments, and participate in extracurricular activities. She has even refused playdates and outings unless her mother can be present.

Previous Interventions or Diagnoses:

Mia has not received any formal mental health treatment prior to the onset of her symptoms. Her parents have attempted to reassure her and provide emotional support, but they are increasingly concerned about the impact her anxiety is having on her schooling and social life. They have reached out to a clinician for guidance on how best to support Mia.

Clinical Decision-Making Process

DSM-5-TR Diagnostic Criteria Considered:
- **Developmentally Inappropriate and Excessive Anxiety about Separation**: According to the DSM-5-TR, Separation Anxiety Disorder involves excessive anxiety concerning separation from home or from attachment figures. Mia's intense worry about being separated from her mother and her physical symptoms align with this criterion.

- **Duration and Impact on Daily Functioning**: Mia's symptoms have persisted for over a year and interfere with her ability to attend school, socialize, and participate in typical childhood activities, fulfilling the DSM-5-TR requirement for functional impairment.

- **Persistent Worry and Refusal to Be Alone**: Mia frequently expresses fears about her mother's safety and refuses to stay alone or be without her mother, particularly at night. This persistent worry and behavioral avoidance further support the diagnosis of Separation Anxiety Disorder.

Exclusion of Other Diagnoses:
- **Generalized Anxiety Disorder (GAD)**: While Mia does experience anxiety, her worry is specific to separation from her family members rather than generalized across various life areas, ruling out GAD.

- **Social Anxiety Disorder**: Although Mia avoids certain situations, her avoidance is motivated by fear of separation rather than fear of social judgment or embarrassment, differentiating her symptoms from Social Anxiety Disorder.

- **Specific Phobia**: Mia's anxiety is not associated with a specific object or situation, but rather a pervasive fear of separation from her loved ones, distinguishing it from specific phobias.

Assessment Tools:
- **Separation Anxiety Scale for Children (SASC)**: This tool assessed Mia's level of anxiety related to separation, confirming a high degree of anxiety that affects her daily functioning.

- **Multidimensional Anxiety Scale for Children (MASC)**: The MASC provided additional insight into the severity of Mia's anxiety symptoms, particularly in relation to her physical symptoms and fears of harm, supporting the diagnosis.

- **Clinical Interview with Family**: A structured interview was conducted with Mia and her parents to understand her attachment behaviors, worries, and impact on daily life, confirming that her symptoms align with the DSM-5-TR criteria for Separation Anxiety Disorder.

Family Discussion: The clinician met with Mia's parents to discuss the diagnosis of Separation Anxiety Disorder and how it affects Mia's development and daily life. The clinician recommended a combination of cognitive-behavioral therapy (CBT) and gradual exposure techniques to help Mia address her fears and increase her independence. Psychoeducation was provided to Mia's parents to help them understand the importance of supporting Mia's gradual separation while avoiding over-reassurance. The clinician also recommended regular check-ins and family sessions to support Mia's progress.

Suggested Topics
- Cognitive-behavioral therapy and gradual exposure for Separation Anxiety Disorder.
- Differentiating Separation Anxiety Disorder from other anxiety disorders in children.
- The role of family support and strategies for fostering independence in children with separation anxiety.

Chapter 18: **Clinical Cases in Trauma- and Stressor-Related Disorders**

18.0 Introduction to Trauma- and Stressor-Related Disorders

Trauma- and stressor-related disorders encompass a group of mental health conditions that arise following exposure to a traumatic or stressful event. Unlike other disorders, these conditions are unique in that they require the presence of a distressing life event as a diagnostic criterion. The nature, severity, and timing of the traumatic experience are integral to understanding how symptoms develop and persist. While some individuals may exhibit resilience after experiencing trauma, others may develop significant psychological symptoms that affect their daily functioning, relationships, and quality of life.

The DSM-5-TR categorizes trauma- and stressor-related disorders into specific types, each with distinct diagnostic criteria and symptom patterns. Post-Traumatic Stress Disorder (PTSD) is characterized by intrusive memories, avoidance behaviors, and heightened arousal following a traumatic event, such as physical violence or natural disaster. Acute Stress Disorder shares similar symptoms to PTSD but occurs within a shorter time frame following the trauma. Adjustment Disorder involves emotional or behavioral symptoms in response to a significant life change or stressor, though the response is less intense than in PTSD. Reactive Attachment Disorder and Disinhibited Social Engagement Disorder are both typically seen in children with a history of severe neglect, affecting their attachment and social behaviors. Lastly, Trauma-Induced Dissociative Disorder can manifest as a disruption in memory, consciousness, identity, or perception, often as a psychological defense against overwhelming trauma.

These disorders frequently involve complex interactions between psychological, biological, and social factors. Treatment often requires a multi-modal approach, including psychotherapy, psychoeducation, and sometimes medication, to address both immediate symptoms and underlying trauma. Understanding the nuances of each disorder within this category is essential for clinicians and students, as they explore various cases in this chapter to deepen their knowledge of trauma-informed care and evidence-based treatment options for those impacted by trauma and stressor-related disorders.

Case 18.1: Post-Traumatic Stress Disorder (PTSD)

Patient Presentation
Patient: Sarah, a 29-year-old female

Family Background: Sarah is a married mother of one child, a three-year-old daughter. She and her husband live in an urban area, where she works as an elementary school teacher. Six months ago, Sarah was involved in a severe car accident while driving home from work. Although she sustained only minor physical injuries, the incident was traumatic, with her car spinning out of control after being hit by a large vehicle. Since then, Sarah's family has observed significant changes in her mood, behavior, and daily functioning.

Key Symptoms:
- **Intrusive Memories and Flashbacks**: Sarah experiences frequent, involuntary flashbacks and vivid memories of the accident, often triggered by sounds like screeching brakes or loud traffic. She reports feeling as though she is "back in the car" during these episodes, which cause intense distress.

- **Avoidance Behavior**: She avoids driving altogether and refuses to go near the intersection where the accident occurred. Her husband now drives her to work, but she remains visibly anxious in the car, often closing her eyes during the trip to avoid looking at the road.

- **Hyperarousal and Irritability**: Sarah has become easily startled, particularly by sudden noises, and frequently scans her environment for potential dangers. She is noticeably irritable, and her family reports that she often snaps at them over minor issues.

- **Negative Mood and Cognitive Changes**: Sarah feels detached from her friends and family and has developed a sense of hopelessness about the future. She believes she will never feel safe in a car again and expresses guilt, feeling that she "should have been able to avoid the accident."

Symptom Evolution:

Sarah's symptoms emerged soon after the accident and have worsened over time. Initially, she attributed her anxiety to general nerves, but as her intrusive memories and flashbacks became more frequent, she began avoiding more activities and situations related to driving. Her husband reports that she has become distant, spending less time with family and engaging less with their child. Sarah's distress has led her to consider taking a leave from her teaching position due to her ongoing anxiety and fear of leaving the house.

Previous Interventions or Diagnoses:

Sarah has not received any formal mental health treatment before the accident. She attempted to manage her symptoms independently, hoping that her anxiety would subside with time. However, as her symptoms persisted and began to interfere significantly with her life, her family encouraged her to seek professional help.

Clinical Decision-Making Process

DSM-5-TR Diagnostic Criteria Considered:

- **Exposure to Traumatic Event**: The DSM-5-TR requires direct exposure to a traumatic event as a criterion for PTSD. Sarah's severe car accident, where she believed she might die, qualifies as a traumatic event.

- **Intrusive Symptoms**: Sarah exhibits key intrusive symptoms, including recurrent, involuntary memories of the accident, flashbacks, and intense distress upon exposure to triggers like traffic sounds. These meet the DSM-5-TR criteria for PTSD.

- **Avoidance**: Her avoidance of driving, reluctance to approach the accident site, and attempts to suppress her memories fulfill the DSM-5-TR avoidance criterion.

- **Negative Alterations in Cognition and Mood**: Sarah's feelings of detachment, persistent negative beliefs about her safety, and guilt are consistent with the DSM-5-TR's cognitive and mood criteria for PTSD.

- **Arousal and Reactivity**: Sarah's hypervigilance, exaggerated startle response, and irritability fulfill the arousal symptoms required for a PTSD diagnosis.

Exclusion of Other Diagnoses:

- **Acute Stress Disorder**: Although Sarah's symptoms began shortly after the trauma, they have persisted for over six months, ruling out Acute Stress Disorder, which is limited to the first month post-trauma.

- **Generalized Anxiety Disorder (GAD)**: While Sarah experiences anxiety, it is specific to the trauma and related triggers rather than a general, pervasive worry across multiple areas of her life, ruling out GAD.

- **Adjustment Disorder with Anxiety**: Sarah's symptoms are directly tied to the trauma and include flashbacks, avoidance, and hyperarousal, which are more consistent with PTSD than with an adjustment disorder.

Assessment Tools:

- **Clinician-Administered PTSD Scale for DSM-5 (CAPS-5)**: This structured interview tool confirmed the presence and severity of Sarah's PTSD symptoms, providing a comprehensive overview of her distress and functional impairment.

- **PTSD Checklist for DSM-5 (PCL-5)**: The PCL-5 assessed Sarah's PTSD symptoms across DSM-5 criteria, indicating high levels of trauma-related distress.

- **Beck Depression Inventory (BDI-II)**: This tool was used to assess Sarah's mood, confirming the presence of depressive symptoms that often co-occur with PTSD.

Family Discussion: The clinician met with Sarah and her husband to discuss her PTSD diagnosis, the nature of trauma responses, and potential treatment strategies. Sarah was informed about trauma-focused cognitive-behavioral therapy (CBT) and prolonged exposure therapy, both of which have shown effectiveness in treating PTSD. The clinician also discussed the possibility of integrating relaxation techniques and mindfulness exercises to help Sarah manage her hyperarousal symptoms. Sarah's husband was encouraged to provide emotional support, remain patient with her progress, and assist in facilitating her gradual return to driving and other daily activities.

Suggested Topics
- Trauma-focused cognitive-behavioral therapy (CBT) and prolonged exposure therapy for PTSD.
- Understanding the physiological and psychological effects of trauma and how they relate to PTSD symptoms.
- Differentiating PTSD from Acute Stress Disorder and Adjustment Disorder, focusing on symptom persistence and severity.

Case 18.2: Acute Stress Disorder

Patient Presentation
Patient: Emily, a 34-year-old female

Family Background: Emily is married with two young children. She recently experienced a traumatic incident in which she witnessed a serious workplace accident. Emily works as a project manager for a construction company, and two weeks ago, a fellow employee fell from a considerable height on site. Emily was among the first to reach the scene and waited with the injured coworker until emergency responders arrived. Since the incident, she has had noticeable difficulty managing her emotions and has exhibited changes in her behavior, which her husband and colleagues have observed.

Key Symptoms:
- **Intrusive Memories and Flashbacks**: Emily experiences vivid and distressing flashbacks of the accident, often triggered by sounds or visual reminders associated with the construction site. She reports that, at times, she feels as though she is reliving the moment of the incident.

- **Avoidance Behavior**: She has begun avoiding the specific area of the worksite where the accident occurred. Emily also avoids talking about the incident, as doing so brings up overwhelming emotions.

- **Hyperarousal and Startle Response**: Emily reports feeling constantly "on edge" and finds herself reacting strongly to sudden noises, such as loud machinery. She has difficulty relaxing and feels jumpy even at home.
- **Emotional Numbing and Detachment**: Emily describes feeling emotionally numb and disconnected from her loved ones. She struggles to experience positive emotions and often feels indifferent, even around her children.

Symptom Evolution:

Emily's symptoms began almost immediately after the traumatic incident. She initially dismissed her reactions as temporary but has become increasingly concerned as her symptoms persist and interfere with her ability to function at work and at home. Although she wants to support her coworker's recovery, she finds it too distressing to discuss the accident, leading her to withdraw from both work-related and social discussions.

Previous Interventions or Diagnoses:

Emily has no prior history of mental health issues and has not previously sought psychiatric care. Her family encouraged her to speak with a mental health professional as her symptoms began to affect her daily functioning and relationships.

Clinical Decision-Making Process

DSM-5-TR Diagnostic Criteria Considered:
- **Exposure to Traumatic Event**: The DSM-5-TR specifies that Acute Stress Disorder can be diagnosed after an individual experiences or witnesses a traumatic event. Emily's direct exposure to a life-threatening incident involving her coworker qualifies as a traumatic experience.

- **Intrusive Symptoms**: Emily's recurrent and distressing flashbacks, combined with her reliving of the incident, meet the DSM-5-TR criteria for intrusive symptoms in Acute Stress Disorder.

- **Avoidance**: Emily's avoidance of the accident site and reluctance to discuss the incident align with the avoidance criteria required for Acute Stress Disorder.

- **Negative Mood and Dissociation**: Emily's feelings of emotional numbness and detachment, as well as her inability to feel positive emotions, meet the mood and dissociative criteria for Acute Stress Disorder.

- **Arousal and Hypervigilance**: Emily's hypervigilance, heightened startle response, and difficulty relaxing further confirm the arousal symptoms required for this diagnosis.

Exclusion of Other Diagnoses:
- **Post-Traumatic Stress Disorder (PTSD)**: Although Emily's symptoms are consistent with a trauma response, her symptoms have been present for less than a month, which aligns with the time frame for Acute Stress Disorder rather than PTSD. A diagnosis of PTSD requires symptoms to persist for more than a month.

- **Adjustment Disorder with Anxiety**: Emily's symptoms are specifically tied to a traumatic event, rather than to a general life stressor, and include trauma-specific symptoms like flashbacks and hypervigilance, which differentiate her symptoms from an adjustment disorder.

Assessment Tools:
- **Acute Stress Disorder Interview (ASDI)**: This interview-based tool confirmed the presence of specific symptoms of Acute Stress Disorder, allowing the clinician to assess symptom frequency, severity, and impact on functioning.

- **Impact of Event Scale-Revised (IES-R)**: The IES-R assessed the intensity of Emily's trauma-related symptoms, such as intrusion, avoidance, and hyperarousal, supporting the diagnosis.

- **Clinical Interview**: A structured interview helped clarify the nature and progression of Emily's symptoms, confirming that they meet the DSM-5-TR criteria for Acute Stress Disorder.

Family Discussion: The clinician met with Emily and her husband to discuss her diagnosis and explain the typical course of Acute Stress Disorder. Psychoeducation was provided to help Emily and her family understand that many people experience strong reactions to trauma, and that these reactions often improve with supportive care and treatment. Treatment options, including trauma-focused cognitive-behavioral therapy (CBT) and relaxation techniques, were discussed to help Emily process the trauma and reduce her arousal symptoms. Emily's husband was encouraged to provide emotional support and create a calming environment at home, facilitating Emily's recovery.

Suggested Topics
- Understanding the timeline and symptom criteria distinguishing Acute Stress Disorder from PTSD.
- Trauma-focused cognitive-behavioral therapy (CBT) techniques for Acute Stress Disorder.
- The role of family and social support in the early stages of trauma recovery.

Case 18.3: Adjustment Disorder

Patient Presentation
Patient: Michael, a 45-year-old male

Family Background: Michael lives with his wife and two teenage children in a suburban area. He recently lost his job of 15 years due to company downsizing. This sudden change has significantly impacted his financial stability and self-esteem. Michael has always prided himself on being the primary provider for his family and finds himself struggling to adjust to his new reality, feeling increasingly overwhelmed and anxious about his future.

Key Symptoms:
- **Anxiety and Worry**: Michael reports feeling excessively worried about his financial situation and future job prospects. He spends hours each day searching for jobs online and becomes highly anxious whenever he thinks about his family's financial stability.

- **Depressed Mood**: He frequently feels down and defeated, expressing that he "failed" his family by not being able to secure another job quickly. Michael's self-esteem has been significantly impacted, and he finds himself dwelling on negative thoughts about his self-worth.

- **Irritability and Withdrawal**: Michael has become more irritable with his family members, often withdrawing to his room to avoid social interaction. He feels guilty for being unable to engage in family activities and worries about being a burden.

- **Sleep Disruption**: His anxiety and ruminative thoughts about his job loss keep him awake at night, resulting in poor sleep quality and fatigue throughout the day.

Symptom Evolution:

Michael's symptoms began shortly after he was laid off from his job two months ago. Initially, he experienced mild stress and worry, but as he struggled to secure new employment, his anxiety and low mood intensified. He now finds it difficult to maintain his usual daily routine, with his anxiety and depressive symptoms interfering with his ability to care for himself and connect with his family. His family encouraged him to seek help after noticing his withdrawal and persistent distress.

Previous Interventions or Diagnoses:

Michael has no history of mental health treatment or previous psychiatric diagnoses. He has typically been resilient in facing life's challenges, but the sudden loss of his job has triggered an emotional response he feels unable to manage independently.

Clinical Decision-Making Process

DSM-5-TR Diagnostic Criteria Considered:
- **Presence of an Identifiable Stressor**: According to the DSM-5-TR, Adjustment Disorder is diagnosed when an individual experiences emotional or behavioral symptoms in response to a specific stressor within three months of its onset. Michael's job loss serves as a clear and identifiable stressor that precipitated his symptoms.

- **Significant Impairment in Functioning**: Michael's worry, irritability, and depressive symptoms interfere with his daily life and social relationships, fulfilling the DSM-5-TR requirement for functional impairment.

- **Symptoms Not Meeting Criteria for Other Disorders**: His symptoms do not meet the threshold for a Major Depressive Disorder or Generalized Anxiety Disorder, as they are directly tied to a specific stressor and do not include the full range of criteria for those conditions.

Exclusion of Other Diagnoses:
- **Major Depressive Disorder (MDD)**: Although Michael exhibits some depressive symptoms, his symptoms are specifically tied to the recent stressor of job loss and are not pervasive across multiple areas of his life, ruling out MDD.

- **Generalized Anxiety Disorder (GAD)**: While Michael experiences anxiety, it is centered on his current life situation rather than a generalized worry across various domains, helping differentiate his symptoms from GAD.

- **Acute Stress Disorder**: Michael's symptoms are tied to a stressor rather than a traumatic event, and he does not exhibit the intrusive or dissociative symptoms characteristic of Acute Stress Disorder.

Assessment Tools:
- **Adjustment Disorder New Module (ADNM)**: This tool evaluated the severity and impact of Michael's symptoms, confirming a level of stress and impairment consistent with Adjustment Disorder.

- **Beck Depression Inventory-II (BDI-II)**: The BDI-II assessed the presence and severity of Michael's depressive symptoms, supporting a moderate level of mood disturbance in relation to his recent stressor.

- **Clinical Interview**: A structured interview helped clarify Michael's symptoms and responses to the stressor, confirming that his experiences align with DSM-5-TR criteria for Adjustment Disorder.

Family Discussion: The clinician met with Michael and his wife to discuss the diagnosis of Adjustment Disorder and the normalcy of such responses following a significant life change. Psychoeducation was provided to both Michael and his wife, explaining that while distress is expected, supportive measures can promote resilience and improve his adjustment process. Treatment options, including solution-focused therapy and cognitive-behavioral therapy (CBT), were discussed to help Michael develop coping strategies and manage his anxiety. His family was encouraged to provide a supportive environment, avoiding any undue pressure while Michael navigates this transitional period.

Suggested Topics
- Solution-focused therapy and cognitive-behavioral techniques for managing Adjustment Disorder.
- Understanding the distinction between Adjustment Disorder and other mood and anxiety disorders.
- Coping strategies for navigating significant life changes, with a focus on resilience-building.

Case 18.4: Reactive Attachment Disorder

Patient Presentation

Patient: Liam, a 6-year-old male

Family Background: Liam was adopted by his current family at the age of 4, after spending his first years in an overcrowded orphanage with minimal caregiver attention. His adoptive parents report that, since joining their family, Liam has struggled to form a close bond with them and often displays unusual social behaviors for his age. Although they have provided him with a stable, nurturing environment, they are concerned about his emotional responses and difficulty connecting with others.

Key Symptoms:

- **Emotional Withdrawal**: Liam appears emotionally distant and rarely seeks comfort from his parents, even when he is upset or injured. He often responds passively to affection, showing minimal emotional reciprocity.

- **Limited Positive Affect**: His parents observe that Liam rarely displays joy, enthusiasm, or other positive emotions. When playing or engaging in activities, he seems indifferent, without the typical excitement children his age express.

- **Unexplained Irritability and Sadness**: Liam often appears irritable and occasionally exhibits prolonged episodes of sadness without a clear cause. His parents report that he is quick to become frustrated and sometimes reacts to minor challenges with unexpected anger or withdrawal.

- **Difficulty Forming Relationships**: In social settings, Liam shows little interest in interacting with other children or adults. He neither actively seeks out relationships nor responds positively when approached, making it difficult for him to develop friendships or close bonds.

Symptom Evolution:

Liam's symptoms have been present since his adoptive parents first brought him home, though they initially attributed them to the stress of adjusting to a new environment. Over time, however, they noticed that he was not responding to their affection or efforts to engage him as expected. His behaviors have remained consistent over the past two years, and despite their attempts to provide him with love and attention, Liam continues to struggle with emotional and social connections.

Previous Interventions or Diagnoses:

Prior to his adoption, Liam had limited exposure to consistent caregiving, which is documented in his orphanage records. His adoptive parents have worked with pediatricians and behavioral specialists to address his social and emotional challenges, but no formal diagnosis was made until now.

Clinical Decision-Making Process

DSM-5-TR Diagnostic Criteria Considered:
- **History of Insufficient Care**: The DSM-5-TR specifies that Reactive Attachment Disorder (RAD) arises in children who have experienced neglect or a lack of stable caregiving in early life. Liam's history of being raised in an institution with limited caregiver interaction fulfills this criterion.

- **Consistent Patterns of Emotional Withdrawal**: Liam displays a persistent reluctance to seek comfort from caregivers, even in situations where reassurance is typically needed. His lack of emotional responsiveness and detachment align with the DSM-5-TR criteria for RAD.

- **Minimal Social and Emotional Responsiveness**: Liam's limited display of positive emotions and his tendency toward irritability and sadness support the criteria for emotional and social impairment associated with RAD.

- **Diagnosis Before Age 5**: Although Liam was formally diagnosed at age 6, his symptoms and relevant history align with patterns that have been present since infancy, meeting the DSM-5-TR requirement that RAD symptoms be evident before age 5.

Exclusion of Other Diagnoses:
- **Autism Spectrum Disorder (ASD)**: Although some of Liam's behaviors might resemble those seen in ASD, such as limited social interaction, he does not display the stereotyped behaviors, communication delays, or restricted interests typical of autism. His symptoms are more closely linked to his early deprivation and neglect.

- **Social Anxiety Disorder**: Liam's reluctance to engage socially is related to his attachment style and early caregiving experiences, rather than to an excessive fear of judgment or social scrutiny, differentiating his case from social anxiety.

- **Depressive Disorders**: While Liam exhibits some signs of irritability and sadness, his overall symptoms are more focused on attachment and social responsiveness rather than a pervasive low mood, ruling out a primary diagnosis of a depressive disorder.

Assessment Tools:
- **Attachment-Based Assessment for RAD**: This assessment was used to evaluate Liam's attachment behaviors and responsiveness to caregivers, providing insights into his social withdrawal and emotional detachment.

- **Child Behavior Checklist (CBCL)**: The CBCL was used to assess Liam's behavioral and emotional functioning, identifying key areas of difficulty in social engagement and emotional regulation.

- **Clinical Observations and Parent Interviews**: Through observations and interviews with Liam's parents, the clinician was able to better understand his behavior patterns and emotional responses, confirming that his experiences align with the DSM-5-TR criteria for Reactive Attachment Disorder.

Family Discussion: The clinician met with Liam's adoptive parents to discuss the diagnosis of Reactive Attachment Disorder, explaining how early neglect and lack of caregiver interaction can impact a child's attachment style. Treatment options, including attachment-focused therapy and play therapy, were recommended to help Liam develop trust and emotional connections. The clinician provided psychoeducation on the importance of patience, consistency, and structured routines to support Liam's emotional growth. His parents were encouraged to work closely with therapists and use positive reinforcement to gradually build Liam's capacity for secure attachment.

Suggested Topics
- Attachment-focused therapy and play therapy techniques for Reactive Attachment Disorder.
- Understanding the role of early caregiving and its impact on attachment and emotional development.
- Differentiating Reactive Attachment Disorder from Autism Spectrum Disorder and Social Anxiety Disorder.

Case 18.5: Trauma-Induced Dissociative Disorder

Patient Presentation
Patient: Olivia, a 26-year-old female

Family Background: Olivia lives alone and works as a nurse in a busy urban hospital. She has a close but somewhat strained relationship with her family, as they live in another state and have limited awareness of her recent struggles. Over the past few years, Olivia has experienced multiple traumatic events, including a serious car accident and, more recently, an assault. Since the assault, she has been exhibiting dissociative symptoms that interfere with her daily life and professional responsibilities.

Key Symptoms:
- **Episodes of Dissociation**: Olivia describes frequent episodes of feeling detached from her surroundings, as if she were observing herself from outside her body. These episodes occur unpredictably, often triggered by sudden loud noises or specific smells that remind her of the assault.

- **Memory Gaps and Amnesia**: She reports difficulty remembering specific details of the assault and other stressful events. In some cases, she struggles to recall entire conversations or moments from her day, creating issues at work where she cannot remember patient interactions or important tasks.

- **Emotional Numbing and Detachment**: Olivia feels emotionally distant, both from herself and from others, even close friends and family. She describes feeling as though she is "numb" and finds it difficult to experience joy or empathy, which impacts her work as a caregiver.

- **Increased Stress and Startle Response**: Olivia is highly sensitive to stress and startles easily, especially in situations where she feels vulnerable. Her heightened anxiety and hypervigilance exacerbate her dissociative symptoms, causing her to retreat further from social and work responsibilities.

Symptom Evolution:

Olivia's dissociative symptoms began shortly after the assault, intensifying over the past six months. Initially, she attributed her emotional numbness and memory lapses to the stress of her job, but as her symptoms grew more persistent and intrusive, she recognized that they were affecting her ability to function. Her supervisor at work has noted her inconsistent performance and suggested she seek help after observing her inability to recall basic tasks.

Previous Interventions or Diagnoses:

Olivia had not sought psychological treatment prior to the assault. However, she has struggled with symptoms of anxiety and low mood since the car accident a few years ago. After the assault, her dissociative symptoms became more pronounced, and she eventually sought professional support to help manage her daily functioning.

Clinical Decision-Making Process

DSM-5-TR Diagnostic Criteria Considered:
- **Exposure to Trauma**: Trauma-Induced Dissociative Disorder is characterized by dissociative symptoms following exposure to traumatic events. Olivia's recent assault and previous car accident qualify as traumatic experiences that could trigger dissociation.

- **Symptoms of Depersonalization and Derealization**: Olivia's experiences of detachment, feeling as if she is outside her own body, and emotional numbness meet the DSM-5-TR criteria for depersonalization and derealization associated with dissociative disorders.

- **Memory Impairment**: Her frequent memory lapses and amnesia for traumatic events further support the DSM-5-TR criteria, indicating significant dissociation that impairs her ability to function.

- **Functional Impairment**: Olivia's dissociative symptoms interfere with her daily functioning, affecting her work performance, personal relationships, and overall quality of life, which meets the DSM-5-TR criterion for functional impairment in trauma-induced dissociative disorders.

Exclusion of Other Diagnoses:
- **Post-Traumatic Stress Disorder (PTSD)**: Although Olivia's symptoms overlap with PTSD, her primary symptoms involve depersonalization, derealization, and memory gaps, which are more characteristic of a dissociative disorder than PTSD.

- **Dissociative Identity Disorder (DID)**: Olivia does not report distinct identity states or personalities that would indicate DID, differentiating her presentation as a trauma-induced dissociative disorder.

- **Depressive and Anxiety Disorders**: While Olivia exhibits symptoms of anxiety and emotional numbness, her dissociative experiences, including depersonalization and memory gaps, are not fully explained by mood or anxiety disorders, supporting the diagnosis of a dissociative disorder.

Assessment Tools:
- **Dissociative Experiences Scale (DES)**: This assessment provided a measure of Olivia's dissociative symptoms, including depersonalization, derealization, and amnesia, confirming the presence and severity of her dissociation.

- **Clinician-Administered PTSD Scale (CAPS-5)**: The CAPS-5 assessed her trauma-related symptoms and ruled out a primary diagnosis of PTSD, as her primary symptoms were dissociative in nature.

- **Structured Clinical Interview for DSM-5 Dissociative Disorders (SCID-D)**: This interview-based tool allowed for a comprehensive evaluation of Olivia's dissociative symptoms, further clarifying her experiences of memory lapses and detachment from reality.

Family Discussion: Since Olivia lives independently, the clinician encouraged her to communicate her diagnosis with close family members or trusted friends to build a support system. Psychoeducation was provided to help Olivia understand the nature of trauma-induced dissociation and how it can affect her perception, memory, and emotional responses. Treatment options, including trauma-focused cognitive-behavioral therapy (CBT) and grounding techniques, were discussed to help her manage symptoms in triggering situations. The clinician also recommended gradual re-engagement in social and recreational activities to support her sense of reality and emotional connection.

Suggested Topics
- Trauma-focused therapy and grounding techniques for managing dissociative symptoms.
- Differentiating Trauma-Induced Dissociative Disorder from PTSD and Dissociative Identity Disorder.
- Understanding the impact of trauma on memory, perception, and emotional regulation.

Section 4:
Practical Diagnostic Guides and Quick Reference Tools

Introduction to Section 4

In clinical practice, the accuracy and precision of diagnosis are foundational to effective patient care, guiding both treatment plans and therapeutic outcomes. This section aims to provide practical diagnostic guides and reference tools specifically crafted to enhance your decision-making skills in complex cases. Whether you're working with co-occurring conditions, discerning between overlapping symptoms, or assessing functional impairments, these tools are designed to streamline your diagnostic process, promoting clarity and confidence.

Diagnostic guides in this section offer structured approaches to evaluating complex cases, helping you to methodically assess symptom severity and make informed diagnostic decisions. In scenarios where multiple disorders present together, where patient histories are intricate, or where symptoms are ambiguous, these guides provide a step-by-step framework to approach each case systematically. This section also introduces quick reference tools, such as symptom overlap tables, decision trees, and diagnostic algorithms, which allow you to quickly differentiate between similar conditions and minimize the risk of common diagnostic errors.

Additionally, you'll find resources on assessment tools and rating scales, which serve as valuable metrics for quantifying symptom intensity, evaluating quality of life, and interpreting cultural factors in assessments. These tools not only support more accurate diagnosis but also empower you to monitor progress over time, tailor treatment approaches, and ensure that each patient's unique background is considered.

As you engage with these resources, remember that they are here to reinforce your clinical intuition, improve diagnostic consistency, and provide a solid foundation for navigating even the most challenging cases. Through using these tools, you can streamline the diagnostic process, reduce uncertainty, and ultimately deliver more effective, compassionate care.

Chapter 19: Diagnostic Guides for Complex Cases

19.1 Diagnostic and Management Approaches for Comorbid Disorders

Comorbid disorders, where two or more distinct diagnoses co-occur, present unique challenges in clinical practice, often complicating both the diagnostic process and treatment planning. This section provides a structured approach for identifying and managing comorbid conditions, focusing on how to prioritize diagnostic criteria, balance treatment needs, and develop a coherent management plan that respects the complexities of multiple, overlapping symptoms.

When approaching a case with potential comorbidities, it's essential to begin with a **comprehensive assessment** that captures the full scope of the patient's symptoms, history, and functional impairments. Use this opportunity to identify the primary disorder—often the one most impairing or persistent—and then consider additional diagnoses that may influence or interact with it. For example, in cases where anxiety and depression are both present, identifying which symptoms are most pervasive can help clarify the primary diagnosis and shape subsequent treatment.

A structured diagnostic approach involves using the **DSM-5-TR criteria for each disorder independently** while keeping a holistic view of how symptoms may interact. When assessing for comorbidities, it's beneficial to employ symptom checklists and structured interviews that allow for side-by-side comparison of diagnostic criteria, reducing the likelihood of symptom overlap or diagnostic overshadowing. Additionally, in situations where one disorder may exacerbate another, it is crucial to recognize which symptoms are truly independent of each other versus those that may stem from an overlapping source.

In terms of **management strategies**, balancing the needs of multiple disorders often involves a layered treatment plan. For instance, if treating a patient with both PTSD and a substance use disorder, addressing the substance use may need to precede trauma-focused work, allowing the patient to stabilize before processing traumatic experiences. Similarly, certain therapeutic interventions, like cognitive-behavioral therapy (CBT), can be adapted to address multiple diagnoses by targeting core symptoms that are common across disorders, such as emotional regulation or avoidance behaviors.

When creating a treatment plan, prioritize **collaborative goal setting** with the patient, focusing on realistic, manageable goals for each disorder. Encourage open discussions about symptom interaction, treatment preferences, and potential challenges. Monitoring and adjusting the treatment plan over time is critical, as symptoms from one disorder may fluctuate and affect the course of another.

By following these diagnostic and management approaches, clinicians can navigate the complexities of comorbid disorders with confidence, offering a nuanced, individualized approach that considers the interplay of multiple conditions. This process not only enhances diagnostic accuracy but also fosters a more resilient therapeutic relationship, supporting the patient's progress across all areas of their mental health.

19.2 Evaluating Symptom Severity

Evaluating the severity of symptoms is a critical component of accurate diagnosis and effective treatment planning. By assessing the intensity and functional impact of a patient's symptoms, clinicians gain essential insights into the disorder's progression, the urgency of intervention, and the appropriateness of specific treatment approaches. This section presents various tools and metrics for measuring symptom severity across a range of disorders, along with guidelines on when and how to implement these assessments in clinical practice.

Understanding the Role of Severity in Diagnosis and Treatment

Symptom severity informs both the diagnostic process and the selection of treatment strategies. For example, the DSM-5-TR criteria for some disorders, such as Major Depressive Disorder and PTSD, include specific guidelines for determining severity based on symptom frequency, duration, and impact on functioning. Recognizing severity helps in distinguishing between subclinical symptoms and those that warrant formal diagnosis and intervention. Furthermore, it allows for tailored treatment plans: for instance, more intensive interventions may be appropriate for patients experiencing severe symptoms, while those with mild symptoms may benefit from less intensive or shorter-term approaches.

Key Tools and Scales for Severity Assessment

Several standardized scales are commonly used in clinical settings to evaluate symptom severity. Each of these tools is designed to provide a quantitative measure of symptoms, which can be tracked over time to gauge response to treatment and inform adjustments as necessary.

1. **Patient Health Questionnaire-9 (PHQ-9)**

Widely used for assessing the severity of depressive symptoms, the PHQ-9 provides a score that categorizes depression into mild, moderate, or severe levels. This tool is particularly valuable in initial screenings and ongoing assessments, as it helps to monitor symptom fluctuation in response to treatment.

2. **Generalized Anxiety Disorder-7 (GAD-7)**

The GAD-7 is a brief tool for evaluating the severity of generalized anxiety disorder symptoms. By measuring core anxiety symptoms, it helps clinicians determine the appropriate treatment intensity and assess symptom reduction during therapy.

3. **PTSD Checklist for DSM-5 (PCL-5)**

This tool is specific to PTSD and measures symptom severity across DSM-5-TR symptom clusters (intrusion, avoidance, mood alterations, and arousal). The PCL-5 not only assists in diagnosing PTSD but also in tracking symptom changes over time, making it ideal for trauma-focused therapeutic work.

4. **Young Mania Rating Scale (YMRS)**

For assessing the severity of manic episodes in patients with bipolar disorder, the YMRS provides a structured evaluation of symptoms such as elevated mood, hyperactivity, and irritability. Scores from the YMRS can guide decisions regarding medication adjustments and the need for additional supports.

5. **Brief Psychiatric Rating Scale (BPRS)**

Useful for evaluating the severity of symptoms in patients with psychotic disorders, the BPRS assesses a range of symptoms, including anxiety, depression, and hallucinations. This scale allows clinicians to quantify symptom severity in a way that is useful for patients with complex presentations.

6. **Clinician-Administered Dissociative States Scale (CADSS)**

For patients presenting with dissociative symptoms, the CADSS helps quantify the intensity of depersonalization, derealization, and amnesia. This scale is valuable in monitoring symptoms that may fluctuate in response to stress and trauma processing.

Integrating Severity Measures into Clinical Practice

The choice of assessment tool should reflect the specific symptoms and disorders being addressed. When possible, clinicians should integrate multiple tools to capture a comprehensive picture of symptom severity across domains. For example, a patient with co-occurring depression and anxiety may benefit from both the PHQ-9 and the GAD-7, as this allows for precise tracking of both sets of symptoms. Combining data from these tools also helps in establishing baseline measures, setting realistic treatment goals, and facilitating meaningful progress reviews with patients.

Implementing these assessments as part of routine practice involves regular, structured check-ins with patients. **For example, severity measures can be used at intake, at defined intervals during treatment, and when changes in symptoms are reported**. This approach provides a foundation for evidence-based treatment adjustments, as severity scores offer concrete data on how symptoms are responding to interventions. In addition, when tracking severity over time, clinicians gain valuable insights into long-term outcomes, helping to determine whether maintenance treatments are necessary to prevent relapse or if patients are ready for gradual discontinuation of care.

Using Severity Assessments to Inform Treatment Choices

Severity assessments guide treatment intensity and modality selection. For instance:

- **Mild Symptoms**: Patients with mild symptoms may benefit from brief interventions, psychoeducation, and lifestyle modifications, potentially avoiding the need for medication.

- **Moderate Symptoms**: Patients with moderate symptoms often benefit from more structured psychotherapies such as cognitive-behavioral therapy (CBT), possibly combined with medication depending on individual needs.

- **Severe Symptoms**: Severe cases typically require a combination of pharmacotherapy and intensive psychotherapy, and may also involve a higher frequency of clinical sessions or even inpatient care for stabilization.

By consistently applying these tools and interpreting severity in the context of each patient's unique situation, clinicians can make informed decisions that optimize treatment effectiveness and promote patient-centered care.

19.3 Risk Assessment in Complex Cases

In complex clinical cases, risk assessment becomes a crucial element of the diagnostic and treatment planning process, especially when patients present with comorbidities, severe symptoms, or a history of trauma. Risk assessment aims to evaluate the potential for harm to the patient or others, including risks of self-harm, suicidality, aggression, or neglect. This section provides a structured approach to performing comprehensive risk assessments, focusing on identifying key risk factors, utilizing standardized assessment tools, and formulating responsive treatment plans.

Key Components of Risk Assessment

Identifying Risk Factors: Effective risk assessment starts with identifying both static (historical) and dynamic (changing) risk factors. For example:

- **Static risk factors** include past suicide attempts, a history of violence, or childhood trauma. These are often unchangeable but contribute to the overall risk profile.

- **Dynamic risk factors** include current levels of distress, substance use, access to means (e.g., firearms), and recent life stressors. These factors are changeable and may fluctuate, requiring ongoing monitoring.

For patients with complex presentations, the interaction between static and dynamic risk factors often influences overall risk. Clinicians should evaluate how these factors contribute to the patient's mental state and potential for harm, particularly in individuals with comorbid conditions like mood disorders and substance use.

Assessment Tools for Risk Evaluation: Several standardized tools can aid clinicians in quantifying and understanding risk levels. These tools help ensure that assessments are comprehensive and evidence-based:

- **Columbia-Suicide Severity Rating Scale (C-SSRS)**: Widely used to assess suicidal ideation and behavior, the C-SSRS provides a structured way to evaluate current risk, past ideation, and specific plans or intentions.
- **Violence Risk Assessment Tools**: Tools like the Historical-Clinical-Risk Management-20 (HCR-20) are useful for assessing risk in patients with a history of aggression or violent behavior, providing an organized framework to examine potential risk triggers.
- **Brief Psychiatric Rating Scale (BPRS)**: Particularly useful in assessing patients with psychotic symptoms, the BPRS helps gauge severity in areas like hostility, tension, and confusion, which may be relevant in risk evaluation.

Clinical Interviews and Collateral Information: A thorough clinical interview is essential for understanding the patient's subjective experience and gaining insights into their thoughts, feelings, and behavioral intentions. In complex cases, supplementing self-reported information with collateral sources (e.g., family members, caregivers) can be invaluable, especially if the patient's insight is limited or symptoms interfere with self-awareness. Collateral information can provide additional context regarding changes in behavior, recent stressors, and adherence to treatment plans.

Evaluating Protective Factors: Identifying protective factors is as essential as assessing risk factors. Protective factors—such as a supportive social network, a sense of purpose, access to mental health resources, and previous coping skills—can mitigate risk and help clinicians tailor interventions. Encouraging engagement with these factors can serve as a buffer during high-risk periods. For example, patients with strong family support may benefit from family-involved safety planning, while those with strong coping skills may respond well to structured problem-solving interventions.

Dynamic Monitoring and Documentation: In complex cases, risk assessment is not a one-time process; it requires ongoing monitoring and documentation. Risk levels can shift due to situational changes, response to treatment, or other evolving factors. Clinicians should set regular intervals for reassessment, especially following significant life changes, treatment modifications, or increases in symptom severity. Detailed documentation of each risk assessment and any subsequent changes is essential for tracking progress and informing the treatment team.

Developing a Risk Management Plan
Once risk factors are identified, a comprehensive risk management plan can be formulated. This plan should be specific to the patient's unique profile and may include elements such as:

- **Safety Planning**: Collaboratively developing a safety plan with the patient that outlines specific steps to follow if they experience an increase in suicidal thoughts, aggression, or self-harm tendencies. This often includes identifying warning signs, coping strategies, and emergency contacts.

- **Crisis Intervention Strategies**: For high-risk cases, setting up crisis intervention protocols, including immediate access to crisis hotlines, scheduled frequent check-ins, or even temporary hospitalization if necessary, to ensure safety.

- **Targeted Therapeutic Approaches**: Interventions like Dialectical Behavior Therapy (DBT) for individuals at high risk of self-harm or aggression have proven effective in reducing impulsive behaviors and improving emotional regulation.

- **Engaging a Support Network**: Enlisting the support of trusted family members, friends, or caregivers who can assist the patient in monitoring for early warning signs, adhering to treatment, and accessing emergency support if needed.

Case Example: Risk Management in a Patient with Bipolar Disorder and Substance Use

To illustrate, consider a 40-year-old male patient with bipolar disorder and comorbid alcohol use who presents with recent suicidal ideation following a significant life stressor (e.g., job loss). Static risk factors include a history of suicide attempts and long-term alcohol dependency. Dynamic factors include recent mood destabilization and an increase in substance use. Protective factors identified include a supportive family and previous success with mood stabilization medication.

The clinician implements a risk management plan including:
- A detailed safety plan, accessible to both the patient and his spouse, outlining steps to take during episodes of suicidal ideation.
- Frequent follow-up sessions to monitor for changes in mood, substance use, and adherence to treatment.
- Collaborative family involvement in the management plan to enhance adherence to both mood stabilizers and alcohol-reduction goals.

By creating a dynamic and individualized plan, the clinician addresses both immediate and long-term risk factors, providing a structured approach to managing risk in this complex case.

In complex cases, comprehensive risk assessment and management ensure that patients are supported in a structured, proactive way that minimizes potential harm. By using these strategies and tools, clinicians can maintain a high standard of care while navigating the intricate factors that influence risk in patients with co-occurring disorders, severe symptoms, and challenging life circumstances.

Chapter 20: **Differential Diagnosis and Decision-Making Tools**

20.1 Symptom Overlap: Tables and Guides

Symptom overlap between various mental health disorders presents a common challenge in diagnostic accuracy, particularly in cases where conditions share similar presentations. This section provides structured tables and guidelines designed to help clinicians quickly differentiate between disorders with overlapping symptoms. These tools serve as a quick reference for use during assessments, helping to clarify nuanced distinctions and avoid potential misdiagnoses.

Understanding Symptom Overlap in Clinical Practice

Disorders such as anxiety, depression, bipolar disorder, and PTSD often share core symptoms, such as disturbances in sleep, concentration issues, or mood instability. For instance, both Major Depressive Disorder (MDD) and Generalized Anxiety Disorder (GAD) involve feelings of worry, fatigue, and irritability, while bipolar disorder and borderline personality disorder may share mood lability. Without clear differentiation, the clinician risks oversimplifying or misattributing symptoms, which may lead to an ineffective treatment plan.

To address these issues, tables and guides focused on symptom overlap provide a structured approach to assessing symptoms that may appear in multiple disorders. By using these tools, clinicians can evaluate symptoms in a context-specific manner, examining variations in frequency, triggers, and associations with other behavioral patterns.

Examples of Symptom Overlap Tables

The following are examples of tables that could be used to clarify symptom overlap among specific disorders, with a focus on distinguishing between subtle but significant differences.

Table 1: Distinguishing Major Depressive Disorder (MDD) and Generalized Anxiety Disorder (GAD)

Symptom	Major Depressive Disorder (MDD)	Generalized Anxiety Disorder (GAD)
Core Mood Presentation	Persistent sadness or hopelessness	Persistent worry or fear
Primary Triggers	Not necessarily situation-specific; may include internal factors	Often situational or anticipatory
Sleep Disturbances	Insomnia or hypersomnia, often difficulty waking in the morning	Difficulty falling asleep, restlessness related to worry
Cognitive Symptoms	Difficulty concentrating, slow processing	Difficulty concentrating due to pervasive worry
Somatic Complaints	Fatigue, changes in appetite, psychomotor slowing	Muscle tension, restlessness, physical symptoms related to anxiety
Response to Positive Events	Blunted response, little pleasure from positive events	May experience brief relief but returns quickly to worry

This table highlights how shared symptoms, such as sleep disturbances and concentration issues, present differently in each disorder. By focusing on these subtle variations, clinicians can build a clearer picture of which disorder is primary, enabling more targeted interventions.

Table 2: Differentiating Bipolar Disorder and Borderline Personality Disorder (BPD)

Symptom	Bipolar Disorder	Borderline Personality Disorder (BPD)
Mood Instability	Cyclical mood episodes (depression, mania, hypomania)	Rapid mood shifts triggered by interpersonal stressors
Duration of Mood Changes	Episodes lasting days to weeks	Shifts that may last minutes to hours
Impulsivity	Often during manic episodes	Persistent impulsivity in various contexts
Relationship Patterns	May be stable outside mood episodes	Intense and unstable relationships, fear of abandonment
Self-Image	Typically stable outside of mood episodes	Chronic feelings of emptiness and unstable self-image
Risky Behaviors	Primarily during manic or hypomanic episodes	Occurs more frequently and outside specific mood episodes

This table serves as a quick reference to distinguish between bipolar disorder, which is primarily episodic, and BPD, which involves pervasive instability across moods, relationships, and self-image.

Guidelines for Using Symptom Overlap Tables in Practice

1. **Consider Context and Duration**

   Understanding the context in which symptoms appear is essential for distinguishing between overlapping symptoms. For example, mood shifts in BPD are often triggered by relational stress and resolve quickly, while bipolar mood episodes typically last days to weeks.

2. **Assess Symptom Patterns Over Time**

Analyzing symptom patterns over a longer period can clarify whether symptoms are situational (as in PTSD flashbacks) or continuous (as in dissociative disorders). Encourage patients to discuss their history and progression of symptoms to gain a more comprehensive view.

3. **Combine Tables with Structured Interviews**

   Tables are most effective when paired with structured interviews that allow further exploration of symptoms. Use tools like the MINI (Mini International Neuropsychiatric Interview) to probe symptom duration, frequency, and intensity in a standardized format.

4. **Document Observations and Assess Symptom Specificity**

   As you consult symptom tables, document specific observations related to frequency, intensity, and patient descriptions. This documentation can reveal symptom specificity and enhance the accuracy of differential diagnosis.

5. **Evaluate Co-Occurrence of Symptoms**

   If symptoms of multiple disorders are present, consider whether they are truly independent or if one disorder may be primary. For instance, depression secondary to anxiety may exhibit overlapping fatigue and sleep disturbances but should be evaluated in relation to the anxiety itself.

By using these tables and guides as part of a structured approach, clinicians gain a valuable tool for clarifying complex cases where symptoms overlap significantly. The goal is to promote diagnostic accuracy through an organized, comparative method that reduces ambiguity and ensures that each symptom is evaluated in its proper context. This ultimately enhances the quality of care and helps tailor treatment plans that address the specific nuances of each patient's presentation.

20.2 Decision Trees and Diagnostic Algorithms

In complex clinical settings, decision trees and diagnostic algorithms offer a structured approach to differential diagnosis, allowing clinicians to navigate symptom presentations systematically. These tools guide clinicians through a sequence of yes-or-no questions or specific diagnostic checkpoints, helping to rule out less likely conditions while focusing on the most probable diagnosis. In this section, we introduce decision trees and algorithms designed for common clinical scenarios with overlapping or ambiguous symptoms.

The Value of Decision Trees and Diagnostic Algorithms

Decision trees and algorithms provide an efficient framework to evaluate multiple potential diagnoses by simplifying complex symptomatology into sequential decision points. For clinicians facing cases where symptoms cross multiple diagnostic categories—such as mood instability, cognitive impairment, or psychotic features—these tools can help clarify the path toward a definitive diagnosis by reducing diagnostic errors and increasing consistency

Examples of Decision Trees for Differential Diagnosis

Example 1: Decision Tree for Mood Disorders with Psychotic Features

This decision tree aids in differentiating between Major Depressive Disorder with psychotic features, Bipolar Disorder with psychotic features, and Schizoaffective Disorder. It provides clear checkpoints based on symptom duration, mood episode patterns, and the timing of psychotic symptoms relative to mood changes.

Step 1: Are psychotic symptoms present?
- **Yes** → Continue to Step 2.
- **No** → Consider other mood disorders without psychotic features.

Step 2: Is there a history of manic or hypomanic episodes?
- **Yes** → Possible **Bipolar Disorder with psychotic features**; confirm by evaluating mood episode frequency and type.
- **No** → Continue to Step 3.

Step 3. Do psychotic symptoms occur only during mood episodes?
- **Yes** → Possible **Major Depressive Disorder with psychotic features**; confirm by assessing the severity and content of depressive episodes.
- **No** → Consider **Schizoaffective Disorder** if psychotic symptoms occur independently of mood episodes.

This tree emphasizes timing and symptom interaction, crucial factors in distinguishing between mood and psychotic disorders.

Example 2: Decision Tree for Anxiety-Related and Trauma-Related Disorders

This decision tree focuses on distinguishing between Generalized Anxiety Disorder (GAD), Panic Disorder, Social Anxiety Disorder, and Post-Traumatic Stress Disorder (PTSD), particularly in cases where anxiety and avoidance behaviors are prominent.

Step 1. Is anxiety associated with a specific traumatic event?
- Yes → Possible PTSD; evaluate re-experiencing symptoms (e.g., flashbacks, nightmares).
- No → Continue to Step 2.

Step 2. Does the patient experience sudden, unexpected panic attacks?
- Yes → Possible Panic Disorder; assess frequency and impact of panic episodes.
- No → Continue to Step 3.

Step 3. Is anxiety focused on social situations with fear of judgment?
- Yes → Possible Social Anxiety Disorder; confirm by exploring situational triggers.
- No → Consider Generalized Anxiety Disorder if anxiety is pervasive and not situation-specific.

This tree provides checkpoints that emphasize situational triggers and specific symptom patterns associated with each anxiety-related condition.

Diagnostic Algorithms for Complex Cases
Diagnostic algorithms function as step-by-step guides, progressing through layers of symptoms and ruling out specific conditions at each stage. The following examples illustrate how algorithms can be used to manage complex cases involving multiple overlapping symptoms.

Algorithm 1: Differentiating Depressive Symptoms in Medical vs. Psychiatric Contexts

Step 1. Are depressive symptoms chronic or episodic?
- Chronic → Continue to Step 2.
- Episodic → Proceed with evaluation for Major Depressive Disorder or Bipolar Disorder.

Step 2. Is there a known medical condition or substance use that could contribute to symptoms?

- Yes → Consider Depressive Disorder Due to Another Medical Condition or Substance/Medication-Induced Depressive Disorder.
- No → Continue with psychiatric evaluation for primary depressive disorders.

Step 3. Do depressive symptoms improve with medical or lifestyle adjustments?
- Yes → Depression may be secondary to medical or situational factors.
- No → Consider primary depressive disorder, investigate for comorbid psychiatric conditions if necessary.

Algorithm 2: Identifying Primary Diagnosis in Cases with Mood, Anxiety, and Somatic Symptoms

Step 1. Are mood symptoms primary (depression or mania) and persistent?
- Yes → Continue with mood disorder evaluation (e.g., MDD, Bipolar Disorder).

- No → Proceed to Step 2.

Step 2. Are anxiety symptoms pervasive and associated with physical complaints?
- Yes → Consider Generalized Anxiety Disorder or Somatic Symptom Disorder.
- No → Continue to Step 3.

Step 3. Is there a history of trauma or chronic stress contributing to symptoms?
- Yes → Explore for PTSD or Adjustment Disorder.
- No → Evaluate further for primary anxiety or mood disorder based on presenting features.

Using Decision Trees and Algorithms in Clinical Practice

1. **Clarify Symptom Patterns**

   Decision trees and algorithms help clinicians assess the onset, progression, and contextual triggers of symptoms. By clarifying these patterns, clinicians can focus on critical diagnostic criteria and reduce ambiguity in the diagnostic process.

2. **Track and Document the Decision Path**

   Documenting each step in the diagnostic process is essential for cases requiring a detailed rationale, especially when symptoms evolve or shift over time. Consistent documentation allows clinicians to backtrack if symptoms change or new information arises.

3. **Incorporate Patient Input**

   In complex cases, patient input is crucial. Decision trees and algorithms work best when used alongside patient narratives, providing context for each symptom. Engaging patients in the diagnostic process enhances trust and provides deeper insights into symptom presentations.

4. **Adjust Based on Ongoing Assessment**

   Decision trees and algorithms are starting points rather than fixed routes; clinicians should remain flexible. Re-assessment and adjustment are essential, particularly when dealing with disorders like Bipolar Disorder, which may present differently over time or involve periods of remission.

By integrating decision trees and algorithms into clinical practice, clinicians gain a structured, stepwise framework to differentiate between complex, overlapping disorders. These tools not only expedite the diagnostic process but also provide clarity and consistency, allowing clinicians to make informed decisions with greater confidence.

20.3 Strategies for Differential Diagnosis

Differential diagnosis is a critical skill in clinical practice, allowing clinicians to systematically differentiate between disorders with overlapping or ambiguous symptoms. This section outlines practical strategies for conducting a thorough differential diagnosis, including targeted questions to ask during patient interviews, techniques for gathering comprehensive information, and methods for interpreting patient responses to refine diagnostic accuracy.

Key Strategies for Effective Differential Diagnosis

Focused Questioning to Isolate Primary Symptoms: Start by honing in on the patient's primary symptoms and understanding their specific characteristics. Questions should explore symptom duration, triggers, and patterns, which help to clarify distinctions between similar disorders. For example:

- *"How long have you been experiencing these symptoms?"* — This question establishes the duration of the problem, helping to differentiate chronic conditions (e.g., Persistent Depressive Disorder) from episodic conditions (e.g., Major Depressive Disorder).

- *"Are there specific situations or events that seem to make your symptoms worse?"* — Identifying triggers can help distinguish anxiety disorders (e.g., situational anxiety in Social Anxiety Disorder) from trauma responses (e.g., PTSD flashbacks).

Exploring Symptom Onset and Course: Investigating the onset and progression of symptoms provides insight into the underlying disorder. Ask the patient to describe when and how their symptoms first appeared:

- *"Can you recall a time when you didn't experience these symptoms, or did they seem to develop gradually?"*

- *"Has there been a pattern in how your symptoms come and go over time?"*

Gradual onset with persistent, unchanging symptoms may point toward disorders like Generalized Anxiety Disorder, whereas abrupt onset with episodic changes may suggest mood or psychotic disorders. This approach helps narrow down conditions that may present similarly but differ in progression.

Assessing Functional Impact and Impairment: Understanding the functional impact of symptoms is vital for distinguishing disorders with shared symptoms. Questions should focus on the areas of life most affected by the disorder:

- *"How do these symptoms affect your work, school, or relationships?"*

- *"Have you had to make any significant lifestyle adjustments because of your symptoms?"*

Responses indicating pervasive impairment in multiple areas could suggest disorders with a broad impact, like Major Depressive Disorder or Bipolar Disorder, while more targeted impairment might indicate specific anxiety disorders, such as Social Anxiety Disorder.

Evaluating Coping Mechanisms and Patient Insight: Patients often develop coping mechanisms that can offer clues about their disorder. Ask about strategies they use to manage symptoms:

- *"What do you typically do when you feel this way? Do you have any coping methods that seem to help?"*

- *"Do you recognize patterns in how your mood or symptoms change over time?"*

For instance, patients with Obsessive-Compulsive Disorder (OCD) may describe ritualized behaviors as coping mechanisms, while individuals with PTSD might use avoidance strategies. Patient insight into symptom patterns can also indicate conditions like OCD, where insight varies greatly.

Investigating Comorbid Symptoms and Overlap: Comorbidity is common in mental health, and understanding how multiple symptoms interact can help clarify primary versus secondary diagnoses. Use open-ended questions to explore potential overlaps:

- *"Are there other symptoms that seem to occur alongside your primary concerns?"*

- *"Do you experience other physical or mental changes when your main symptoms are at their peak?"*

For example, comorbid anxiety and depression can often exist together, and distinguishing the primary disorder depends on understanding which symptoms are most persistent or impairing. If anxiety appears in multiple forms (general, situational, or trauma-related), this could suggest an anxiety disorder with a secondary depressive component.

Using Structured Interview Techniques

Symptom-Specific Interviews: Structured interviews like the MINI (Mini International Neuropsychiatric Interview) or SCID (Structured Clinical Interview for DSM Disorders) guide the clinician through a sequence of diagnostic questions. These tools are especially helpful for complex cases with symptoms that cross diagnostic boundaries, providing consistency and thoroughness in the assessment.

Exploring Past Treatment and Responses: Understanding previous treatment experiences can inform the current differential diagnosis. Ask questions like:

- *"Have you tried any treatments in the past for these symptoms? How did they work for you?"*

Past responses to medications or therapies provide valuable information. For example, mood stabilizers may have helped someone with bipolar disorder, while SSRIs could have alleviated anxiety in a patient with Generalized Anxiety Disorder. This history can highlight symptoms that may not be fully addressed by the current diagnosis.

Behavioral Observation During Interview: Non-verbal cues, speech patterns, and mannerisms often provide insight into underlying disorders. For example:

- Patients with anxiety may exhibit restlessness, frequent reassurances, or avoidance of eye contact.
- Individuals with manic symptoms might display rapid speech, grandiosity, or impulsiveness.
- Those with psychotic symptoms may have odd mannerisms, gaze aversion, or lack of focus.

Documenting these observations alongside patient responses allows the clinician to synthesize clinical information more effectively, enhancing diagnostic clarity.

Validating Patient Perceptions and Normalizing Experiences: Engaging with empathy and validating the patient's experiences fosters trust, which is crucial for eliciting honest responses. Use statements like:

- *"It's normal for people to feel hesitant talking about these things, but understanding them helps us find the best way to support you."*
- *"Many people go through similar challenges, and I'm here to help you navigate this process."*

This approach encourages patients to share openly, often leading to more accurate symptom descriptions and reducing the risk of overlooking key details.

Practical Application: Case Example of Differential Diagnosis
Imagine a patient who presents with overlapping symptoms of irritability, low mood, and lack of focus. By asking the questions above, you can uncover details such as:

- The onset of symptoms following a stressful life event (suggesting Adjustment Disorder).
- Coping mechanisms centered around avoidance (suggesting Social Anxiety Disorder).
- Persistent daily worry without specific triggers (suggesting Generalized Anxiety Disorder).

By applying these strategies, the clinician gathers a detailed view of the patient's experiences, systematically excluding less likely conditions and refining the diagnosis based on collected data. This targeted approach supports accurate diagnosis, effective treatment planning, and ultimately enhances patient outcomes.

20.4 Common Diagnostic Errors and How to Avoid Them

In clinical practice, accurate diagnosis is essential for effective treatment, yet common diagnostic errors can lead to misdiagnoses that affect patient outcomes. This section outlines frequent diagnostic pitfalls, such as symptom underestimation or overly broad diagnoses, and offers practical strategies to help clinicians refine their diagnostic process. By recognizing these errors and implementing corrective approaches, clinicians can enhance both diagnostic precision and patient care.

1. Error: Overlooking Comorbid Conditions
Description: It's common to identify a primary disorder without recognizing co-occurring conditions, leading to incomplete treatment plans. For example, a patient presenting with anxiety might also have undiagnosed depression, which can remain unaddressed if overlooked.

Prevention Strategy:
- *Thorough Assessment:* Use structured diagnostic interviews that systematically evaluate potential comorbidities. Tools like the SCID or MINI are valuable in assessing for multiple conditions simultaneously.
- *Comprehensive Symptom Review*: Ask open-ended questions about additional symptoms beyond the primary complaint to identify potential comorbidities, such as mood fluctuations in patients with anxiety disorders.

2. Error: Diagnostic Anchoring

Description: Anchoring occurs when a clinician settles on a preliminary diagnosis early in the assessment process and subsequently fails to consider other possibilities. This bias can lead to incorrect diagnoses, especially in complex cases.

Prevention Strategy:
- *Consider Alternative Diagnoses:* Make a habit of listing at least two or three alternative diagnoses when formulating a treatment plan, ensuring that all plausible options are considered.
- *Continuous Re-evaluation*: Periodically review the diagnosis as new information emerges or as the patient progresses through treatment. This helps in refining or adjusting the diagnosis if symptoms change.

3. Error: Symptom Underestimation

Description: Clinicians may underestimate symptom severity or miss subtle signs, particularly in patients who downplay their symptoms or have high-functioning presentations. This underestimation can lead to delayed intervention or inadequate treatment.

Prevention Strategy:
- *Use Standardized Severity Scales:* Tools such as the PHQ-9 for depression or the GAD-7 for anxiety help quantify symptoms, offering a more objective measure of severity.
- *Seek Collateral Information:* When possible, gather information from family members or other care providers who may have a more complete view of the patient's functioning.

4. Error: Overgeneralizing Symptoms to a Single Diagnosis

Description: Overgeneralization involves attributing multiple symptoms to a single disorder, leading to diagnostic oversimplification. For instance, fatigue and concentration issues might be prematurely attributed to depression when they could indicate other conditions, such as a thyroid disorder or chronic fatigue syndrome.

Prevention Strategy:
- *Systematic Symptom Differentiation:* Use symptom overlap tables or decision trees to differentiate between similar symptoms across disorders.
- *Consider Medical Exclusions:* Rule out potential medical causes for psychological symptoms, particularly for physical symptoms like fatigue or sleep issues.

5. Error: Relying Heavily on Patient Self-Report

Description: While self-reported symptoms are crucial for diagnosis, some patients may lack insight into their condition, have memory issues, or underreport symptoms due to stigma. Sole reliance on self-reporting can lead to missed or incorrect diagnoses.

Prevention Strategy:
- *Conduct Behavioral Observations:* During sessions, observe the patient's behavior, speech, and non-verbal cues, which often provide additional context beyond self-report.
- *Utilize Structured Assessments:* Use tools that include collateral information from family or caregivers, especially when evaluating disorders like psychosis or severe mood disorders, where patient insight may be compromised.

6. Error: Underestimating Cultural Factors

Description: Failing to consider cultural influences on symptom presentation can result in misdiagnosis. For example, certain cultures may express emotional distress through physical symptoms rather than verbal descriptions of anxiety or depression.

Prevention Strategy:
- *Cultural Competence Training*: Engage in ongoing education about cultural factors in mental health, including culturally specific presentations and coping mechanisms.
- *Use Culturally Adapted Assessments:* Employ tools that account for cultural differences, such as the DSM-5 Cultural Formulation Interview, which provides structured questions for exploring cultural influences on symptoms.

7. Error: Confirmatory Bias

Description: Confirmatory bias occurs when a clinician looks for evidence to support an initial diagnosis while ignoring contradictory information. This error can lead to overlooking critical symptoms or missing alternative diagnoses.

Prevention Strategy:
- *Challenge Initial Assumptions:* Adopt a mindset that actively questions initial diagnostic impressions. Use language such as, "What else might explain these symptoms?" during case review.
- *Solicit Second Opinions:* Consult with colleagues when in doubt, especially in cases with ambiguous or conflicting symptomology.

8. Error: Misinterpreting Symptom Presentation Due to Medication Effects

Description: Some patients may exhibit symptoms that are side effects of medication (e.g., sedation from antipsychotics, jitteriness from stimulants), leading to confusion with primary symptoms.

Prevention Strategy:

- *Review Medication History:* Carefully examine the patient's current and past medications to assess potential side effects that could mimic or exacerbate psychiatric symptoms.
- *Consult with Pharmacists or Prescribing Physicians:* Collaborate with other healthcare professionals to clarify whether symptoms may be medication-related, especially when treating patients with polypharmacy.

9. Error: Failing to Identify High-Risk Behaviors

Description: In certain cases, high-risk behaviors (e.g., self-harm, substance abuse) may be overlooked, particularly if the patient downplays them. Missing these behaviors can lead to inadequate risk assessment and safety planning.

Prevention Strategy:

- *Directly Address Risk Behaviors:* Regularly ask about high-risk behaviors, even if they aren't immediately apparent. Using risk-specific screening tools, like the C-SSRS for suicide risk, is also beneficial.
- *Monitor High-Risk Symptoms Over Time:* Schedule follow-ups specifically for monitoring high-risk behaviors, noting any changes and adjusting safety plans accordingly.

10. Error: Diagnosing Based on a Single Symptom Cluster

Description: Focusing too narrowly on a single symptom cluster may obscure the broader clinical picture, leading to an incomplete or incorrect diagnosis. For instance, diagnosing solely based on mood symptoms may miss anxiety or cognitive disturbances.

Prevention Strategy:

- *Holistic Assessment*: Take a broad approach, assessing for mood, anxiety, cognitive, and behavioral symptoms. This ensures a comprehensive diagnostic picture, avoiding the error of narrowing too quickly.
- *Review DSM-5-TR Criteria for Differential Diagnosis:* Use DSM-5-TR criteria to compare potential diagnoses and ensure that the full range of symptoms is considered.

By recognizing these common diagnostic errors and implementing targeted strategies to avoid them, clinicians can significantly improve the accuracy and reliability of their diagnoses. These practices not only enhance patient outcomes but also reinforce a consistent, methodical approach to mental health assessment that prioritizes thoroughness and objectivity.

Chapter 21: **Assessment Tools**

21.1 Overview of Clinical Rating Scales

Clinical rating scales are essential tools in mental health assessment, offering a structured way to quantify symptom severity, track patient progress, and support diagnostic decisions. These scales enable clinicians to establish baselines, monitor changes over time, and compare individual cases to population norms. This section provides an overview of widely used rating scales, highlighting their purpose, appropriate contexts for use, and best practices for integrating them into routine clinical assessments.

The Role of Clinical Rating Scales in Diagnosis and Monitoring

Clinical rating scales serve a dual function: they facilitate accurate diagnosis and enable systematic tracking of a patient's progress. By assigning scores to subjective symptoms, these scales convert qualitative experiences into measurable data, which is invaluable for both initial diagnosis and longitudinal assessment. When used consistently, rating scales can reveal trends in symptom improvement or deterioration, helping clinicians adjust treatment plans accordingly. For example, the Beck Depression Inventory (BDI) is effective for diagnosing depression severity, while the Young Mania Rating Scale (YMRS) aids in assessing manic symptoms in bipolar disorder.

Common Clinical Rating Scales and Their Applications

Beck Depression Inventory (BDI)
- Purpose: The BDI is a self-report scale that assesses the severity of depressive symptoms.
- When to Use: Useful for initial assessment of depression and monitoring changes over time. The BDI is particularly helpful in outpatient settings where ongoing symptom tracking is needed.
- Scoring and Interpretation: Scores range from minimal to severe depression. Regular use helps clinicians assess response to therapy and adjust interventions as necessary.

Generalized Anxiety Disorder-7 (GAD-7)
- Purpose: The GAD-7 is a brief self-report tool for screening and assessing the severity of generalized anxiety symptoms.
- When to Use: Ideal for primary care and mental health settings to identify anxiety levels and monitor progress in treatment.
- Scoring and Interpretation: Scores guide clinical decisions from mild to severe anxiety. It's recommended to use this tool alongside broader assessments to capture the full scope of anxiety-related issues.

Young Mania Rating Scale (YMRS)
- Purpose: The YMRS assesses the severity of manic symptoms, useful in diagnosing and monitoring bipolar disorder.
- When to Use: Primarily used for patients with a known or suspected bipolar diagnosis, especially during acute manic episodes or as part of ongoing care.
- Scoring and Interpretation: A clinician-administered scale that allows tracking of symptom severity, helping guide medication adjustments and therapeutic approaches over time.

Brief Psychiatric Rating Scale (BPRS)
- Purpose: The BPRS evaluates a broad range of psychiatric symptoms, including mood, thought disorders, and behavioral changes.
- When to Use: Useful in both inpatient and outpatient settings, especially for patients with complex presentations that may involve psychosis.
- Scoring and Interpretation: The scale's comprehensive nature makes it ideal for assessing overall symptom burden and monitoring a wide range of symptoms during treatment.

Positive and Negative Syndrome Scale (PANSS)
- Purpose: The PANSS is a clinician-administered scale for assessing positive, negative, and general psychopathology symptoms in patients with schizophrenia.
- When to Use: Primarily in the context of schizophrenia and other psychotic disorders, the PANSS offers an in-depth evaluation of symptom clusters.
- Scoring and Interpretation: By differentiating symptom types, the PANSS aids in tailoring interventions to address positive symptoms (e.g., hallucinations) versus negative symptoms (e.g., social withdrawal).

Best Practices for Using Clinical Rating Scales

Choose Scales that Fit the Clinical Context

Select scales that are tailored to the specific diagnostic needs of your patient population. For example, the PHQ-9 is well-suited for primary care settings, while the PANSS is more appropriate in specialized mental health facilities.

Incorporate Scales into Regular Assessments

Integrate rating scales into routine assessments to track patient progress over time. This is especially useful in cases with chronic or fluctuating symptoms, as it allows clinicians to detect subtle changes that may indicate the need for treatment adjustments.

Engage Patients in the Process

When using self-report scales, involve patients in interpreting their results. Reviewing scores together can foster a collaborative treatment relationship, enhance patient insight, and motivate them to participate actively in their care.

Ensure Consistency in Administration

Use the same scale and scoring criteria consistently across assessments to ensure accurate comparisons over time. Consistency is crucial for establishing reliable baselines and evaluating treatment effects.

Interpret Scores with Clinical Judgment

While rating scales provide valuable quantitative data, they should be interpreted within the broader clinical context. Scores are not diagnostic in isolation but should complement a comprehensive assessment, including clinical interviews and behavioral observations.

By integrating clinical rating scales into diagnostic practice, clinicians gain a structured approach to symptom assessment and progress monitoring. These tools, when used thoughtfully, contribute to more objective and tailored patient care, enhancing the clinician's ability to make informed, evidence-based decisions. In the following sections, we will explore additional assessment tools and techniques that further support comprehensive diagnostic evaluations.

21.2 Diagnostic Questionnaires and Self-Report Tools

Diagnostic questionnaires and self-report tools offer clinicians valuable insights by capturing the patient's subjective experience directly. These tools facilitate efficient screening and assessment of various symptoms, allowing patients to articulate their experiences in a structured format. This section reviews commonly used diagnostic questionnaires and self-report tools, explaining their application in clinical settings and their role in supporting informed decision-making.

The Role of Self-Report Tools in Clinical Practice

Self-report tools provide a patient-centered approach to assessment, where the patient's insights into their symptoms and experiences become a foundational part of the diagnostic process. These tools help bridge the gap between subjective experience and clinical evaluation, supporting a more comprehensive understanding of the patient's condition. For disorders such as depression, anxiety, PTSD, and personality disorders, self-report tools allow patients to express symptom severity and frequency in their own terms, contributing to a well-rounded clinical assessment.

Commonly Used Diagnostic Questionnaires and Self-Report Tools

Patient Health Questionnaire-9 (PHQ-9)

- Purpose: A widely used tool for screening and assessing the severity of depression.
- Application: Particularly useful in primary care and outpatient mental health settings to assess initial depressive symptoms and monitor treatment progress.
- Scoring and Interpretation: Patients rate each item based on symptom frequency over the past two weeks. Scores categorize depression severity from minimal to severe, helping clinicians decide on the level of intervention.

Generalized Anxiety Disorder-7 (GAD-7)

- Purpose: A brief self-report measure that assesses symptoms of generalized anxiety disorder.
- Application: Commonly used as an initial screening tool for anxiety, especially in settings where anxiety symptoms are prevalent.
- Scoring and Interpretation: The GAD-7 evaluates how frequently patients experience symptoms like worry, irritability, and restlessness. Scores help clinicians determine if further anxiety-focused assessment or treatment is needed.

Post-Traumatic Stress Disorder Checklist for DSM-5 (PCL-5)

- Purpose: A self-report questionnaire designed to assess PTSD symptoms according to DSM-5 criteria.
- Application: Used in both clinical and research settings, particularly for trauma-exposed populations. Suitable for initial screening, assessing PTSD severity, and tracking symptom changes over time.
- Scoring and Interpretation: Patients respond to items about re-experiencing, avoidance, hyperarousal, and negative cognitions. Scores indicate symptom severity and support PTSD diagnosis or monitor treatment outcomes.

Mood Disorder Questionnaire (MDQ)

- Purpose: A screening tool for bipolar disorder, assessing the presence of manic or hypomanic episodes.
- Application: Often used in psychiatric settings and primary care to identify potential bipolar disorder cases, guiding further evaluation.
- Scoring and Interpretation: The MDQ screens for core symptoms of mania, such as elevated mood, increased energy, and impulsivity, which help differentiate bipolar disorder from other mood disorders.

Obsessive-Compulsive Inventory-Revised (OCI-R)

- Purpose: A self-report inventory assessing symptoms related to obsessive-compulsive disorder (OCD).
- Application: The OCI-R is used to evaluate symptom frequency and severity, often as part of initial OCD diagnosis or for tracking symptom changes over time.
- Scoring and Interpretation: Items assess common OCD domains like washing, checking, and obsessing. Scores reflect symptom burden and guide treatment decisions based on the specific OCD symptoms reported.

Personality Assessment Inventory (PAI)

- Purpose: A comprehensive self-report inventory that assesses various personality traits and psychopathological symptoms.
- Application: Particularly useful for identifying personality disorders and comorbid conditions, often in outpatient and inpatient psychiatric settings.
- Scoring and Interpretation: The PAI provides insight into areas like interpersonal relationships, emotional stability, and specific personality disorder traits, offering valuable context for both diagnosis and treatment planning.

Best Practices for Using Diagnostic Questionnaires and Self-Report Tools

Choose Tools Based on Clinical Goals

Select self-report tools that are most relevant to the presenting symptoms or the goals of the assessment. For instance, in patients with trauma exposure, the PCL-5 may provide a direct measure of PTSD symptoms, while the GAD-7 would be better suited for generalized anxiety.

Review Responses with the Patient

Incorporate questionnaire results into sessions by discussing responses with the patient. This enhances collaborative understanding, allows for clarification of symptoms, and encourages patient engagement in their treatment journey.

Use Self-Report Tools as Screening Rather Than Diagnostic Tools

Remember that self-report questionnaires are valuable for screening and symptom monitoring but are not diagnostic on their own. They should be used alongside clinical interviews, observation, and other assessment methods for a comprehensive picture.

Monitor Changes Over Time

Re-administer self-report tools periodically to track symptom evolution and treatment response. For instance, a reduction in PHQ-9 scores over several sessions indicates improvement in depressive symptoms, signaling that the current treatment approach may be effective.

Address Limitations and Biases

Be mindful that self-report tools can be subject to patient biases, such as underreporting due to stigma or overreporting during times of acute stress. Encourage honest responses and clarify any confusing items to ensure accurate symptom reporting.

By effectively incorporating diagnostic questionnaires and self-report tools, clinicians can gain a more nuanced view of their patients' mental health, supplementing clinical interviews with structured insights into symptom severity, frequency, and functional impact. When used as part of a comprehensive diagnostic process, these tools contribute significantly to developing a personalized, patient-centered approach to mental health care.

21.3 Functional and Quality of Life Assessments

Functional and quality of life assessments play a vital role in understanding the broader impact of mental health disorders on a patient's daily life. Beyond diagnostic criteria and symptom severity, these assessments capture how a disorder affects the individual's social interactions, work or academic performance, physical health, and overall satisfaction with life. This information is essential for clinicians to design effective, holistic treatment plans that address not only symptom reduction but also overall well-being and functioning.

Understanding Functional Assessments

Functional assessments measure how well patients are managing in different areas of life, highlighting any specific challenges they face in meeting personal, social, and professional responsibilities. For example, in disorders like depression or PTSD, functional impairments can manifest as reduced motivation, difficulty concentrating, or social withdrawal, which may not be immediately apparent through symptom checklists alone. By using functional assessments, clinicians gain insight into these areas of life that may need targeted intervention, such as occupational therapy, social skills training, or academic support.

An example of a commonly used functional assessment is the Global Assessment of Functioning (GAF) scale, which rates the overall level of psychological, social, and occupational functioning. The GAF scale provides a global view of how the patient is functioning in day-to-day life, which can be tracked over time to assess treatment progress. Another example is the WHODAS 2.0 (World Health Organization Disability Assessment Schedule), which examines domains such as mobility, self-care, life activities, and participation in society, giving a broad perspective on functioning across different settings.

Quality of Life Assessments and Their Clinical Relevance

While functional assessments focus on ability, quality of life (QoL) assessments focus on well-being, measuring the patient's subjective satisfaction in various life areas. Quality of life assessments can reveal whether a patient's treatment is truly effective in enhancing their life satisfaction, going beyond symptom management to address the patient's emotional and psychological state. For instance, two patients with similar symptom severity may have vastly different quality of life ratings based on personal resilience, social support, or life circumstances.

A frequently used tool in this area is the WHOQOL-BREF, which measures domains such as physical health, psychological well-being, social relationships, and environmental factors. By evaluating these dimensions, clinicians can understand where a patient may require additional support. For example, if a patient scores low in social relationships, integrating group therapy or family counseling could enhance treatment outcomes and improve life satisfaction.

Integrating Functional and Quality of Life Assessments into Clinical Practice

Using functional and quality of life assessments as part of regular clinical practice allows clinicians to approach treatment with a comprehensive, patient-centered perspective. For new patients, these assessments provide baseline data that inform initial treatment planning, setting realistic goals that align with both symptom improvement and life enhancement. For ongoing cases, periodic re-assessment helps clinicians track changes over time, assess treatment efficacy, and make necessary adjustments.

For example, a patient with schizophrenia may initially struggle with social engagement and occupational stability. Over time, with intervention and support, their functioning may improve in these areas, which can be tracked through periodic functional assessments. Concurrently, quality of life measures can indicate improvements in personal satisfaction and social confidence, offering a more complete picture of recovery.

Enhancing Therapeutic Management through Functional and Quality of Life Insights

Functional and quality of life assessments offer actionable insights for therapeutic management by identifying areas of need that may not emerge from diagnostic interviews alone. When functional limitations are present, clinicians can incorporate adjunctive treatments like vocational training, life skills programs, or occupational therapy to address specific deficits. Likewise, if quality of life assessments highlight dissatisfaction in personal relationships, treatment could incorporate family therapy or social skills training to improve the patient's social support network.

By understanding how mental health disorders impact both function and satisfaction, clinicians are better positioned to create tailored, dynamic treatment plans that go beyond symptom relief. This approach ensures that treatment addresses not just the disorder but the patient's overall capacity to lead a fulfilling life. Through these assessments, clinicians are empowered to make informed adjustments that enhance the patient's quality of life and overall functioning, ultimately fostering a more holistic path to recovery.

21.4 Cultural Considerations in Assessments

Cultural considerations in mental health assessments are essential to achieving accurate, respectful, and effective diagnoses, particularly in diverse, multicultural settings. Cultural background shapes how individuals perceive, interpret, and express symptoms, which means that assessments must be adapted to account for these influences. A culturally sensitive approach ensures that clinicians are not only gathering accurate information but also respecting the patient's unique cultural context, leading to a more precise diagnosis and appropriate treatment plan.

The Impact of Culture on Symptom Expression

Culture influences nearly every aspect of mental health, from how symptoms manifest to how individuals seek help. For instance, some cultures might express emotional distress through physical symptoms rather than verbalizing psychological issues. In certain Asian cultures, for example, somatic complaints like headaches or stomach pain may be the primary way individuals express anxiety or depression, while in Western cultures, verbal expressions of sadness or worry are more common.

An effective culturally sensitive assessment takes these differences into account, asking questions that are open-ended and adaptable to the patient's cultural framework. For instance, rather than asking directly about "feeling sad" or "anxious," clinicians might explore broader questions like, "Have you noticed any changes in your health or energy levels recently?" or "Are there things that worry you or cause stress?" These questions allow the patient to describe their experience in culturally relevant terms, which the clinician can then interpret in a diagnostic context.

Key Cultural Assessment Tools and Frameworks

One of the primary tools for cultural assessment is the **Cultural Formulation Interview (CFI)** included in the DSM-5. The CFI provides a structured approach to exploring cultural factors by addressing four key domains:

1. *Cultural Definition of the Problem*: Understanding the patient's perspective on their condition, including any culturally specific explanations for their symptoms.
2. *Cultural Perceptions of Cause, Context, and Support:* Exploring the patient's beliefs about what caused their symptoms and the role of social and environmental factors.
3. *Cultural Factors Affecting Self-Coping and Past Help-Seeking:* Examining how the patient has previously managed symptoms and whether they sought help, either within or outside the medical system.
4. *Cultural Factors Affecting the Clinician-Patient Relationship:* Recognizing how cultural differences between the clinician and patient may impact communication and trust.

Using the CFI as part of the initial assessment encourages a thorough, respectful exploration of the patient's cultural context, helping to identify factors that might otherwise be overlooked.

Addressing Potential Bias in Assessment
Cultural biases in assessment can lead to misunderstandings or misdiagnoses. For example, behaviors that may be interpreted as avoidance or withdrawal in Western contexts could be seen as expressions of respect or humility in other cultures. Clinicians must be vigilant for such biases, regularly reflecting on their own perspectives and seeking cultural competence through continuous learning and awareness.

One practical strategy is to avoid making assumptions based on a patient's cultural background and instead rely on the patient's narrative to guide the assessment. Engaging in active listening and allowing the patient to describe their symptoms without imposing interpretative biases fosters a more accurate understanding of their experience. It is also helpful to consult with cultural liaisons or interpreters familiar with the patient's cultural background when possible, especially for assessments involving patients from unfamiliar cultural groups.

Integrating Cultural Sensitivity into the Diagnostic Process
To integrate cultural sensitivity into diagnostic practices, clinicians can adopt several key strategies:

Flexibility in Assessment Techniques: Adapting assessment tools and language to align with the patient's cultural frame of reference. For example, for patients who may stigmatize mental health issues, it may be helpful to focus initially on physical symptoms.

Contextualizing Diagnostic Criteria: Recognizing that some DSM criteria may not align perfectly with all cultural expressions of mental illness. Clinicians should use diagnostic criteria as a guide but allow for flexibility in interpretation.

Encouraging Family and Community Involvement: In some cultures, mental health is a collective rather than individual experience. Involving family members or community leaders in the assessment process, when appropriate, can provide valuable insights and support.

Acknowledging Linguistic Nuances: Language barriers can complicate assessments. Even when patients speak the clinician's language, certain words or phrases may carry different connotations. Using simple, clear language and seeking clarification when needed can mitigate misunderstandings.

Case Example: Cultural Sensitivity in Practice

Consider a patient from a cultural background where mental health is stigmatized and often expressed through somatic symptoms. The patient reports chronic fatigue, digestive issues, and muscle tension but denies feeling anxious or depressed. A culturally sensitive approach would involve exploring these physical complaints in depth while gently asking questions about life stressors, relationships, and coping mechanisms without pressing for direct admissions of emotional distress. Over time, the clinician may build rapport and uncover underlying anxiety that the patient feels more comfortable expressing once trust is established.

The Benefits of Culturally Informed Assessments

By incorporating cultural considerations into assessments, clinicians not only improve diagnostic accuracy but also build a more supportive therapeutic relationship. Patients feel respected and understood, which can lead to greater engagement in treatment and better outcomes. In addition, a culturally informed approach encourages clinicians to expand their understanding of mental health as a global and multifaceted experience, enriching their practice and enhancing the quality of care they provide.

Culturally sensitive assessments empower clinicians to understand each patient's unique experience of mental health, ensuring that care is respectful, accurate, and aligned with the patient's values and beliefs. As mental health professionals increasingly encounter diverse populations, a commitment to cultural sensitivity is essential for effective, ethical, and inclusive mental health care.

21.5 Interpretation of Assessment Results

Interpreting assessment results effectively is crucial for transforming raw data into meaningful insights that guide diagnosis and treatment planning. While assessment tools provide quantifiable information on symptom severity, functional impact, and quality of life, the clinician's role is to integrate these findings into a coherent understanding of the patient's overall mental health. This section offers guidance on interpreting assessment results, integrating them into diagnostic formulations, and using them to inform treatment strategies and monitor progress.

Synthesizing Assessment Data for Diagnostic Clarity

Assessment results, such as scores from symptom scales or quality of life measures, should not be viewed in isolation but rather as parts of a broader clinical picture. For example, a high score on a depression inventory suggests significant depressive symptoms, but interpreting it alongside information on functioning and quality of life can clarify the impact on daily life and guide decisions about the intensity of care needed.

To synthesize results, begin by identifying patterns across assessments. If both functional assessments and symptom scales indicate severe impairment, this likely signals a need for more intensive interventions. In contrast, a patient with mild symptoms but significant quality of life impairments may benefit from supportive therapies or skills training. Cross-referencing findings from multiple assessments provides a balanced perspective on the patient's current state, reducing the risk of over- or under-estimating symptom severity.

Contextualizing Scores with Clinical Observations

Numbers alone cannot capture the full complexity of a patient's experience. Clinical observations—such as how a patient interacts during sessions, their emotional affect, and non-verbal cues—add essential context to assessment results. For instance, a patient might score low on an anxiety measure yet appear visibly agitated and avoidant during discussions about social interactions, suggesting underreported symptoms.

To ensure accurate interpretation, compare assessment results with clinical observations and the patient's subjective reports. Discrepancies can indicate areas where further investigation is warranted, perhaps by administering additional assessments or exploring factors like stigma, cultural differences, or insight that might influence how the patient responds to assessment items.

Incorporating Assessment Data into Treatment Planning

Assessment results are instrumental in shaping individualized treatment strategies. High symptom scores, for instance, suggest a need for active symptom management through psychotherapy, medication, or a combination of both. Functional assessments can help prioritize which areas to address in therapy—such as work, relationships, or daily living skills—based on where the patient faces the most challenges.

For patients with chronic conditions, such as bipolar disorder or schizophrenia, interpreting assessment results over time allows clinicians to tailor interventions to current needs. If a patient shows improvement in symptom scores but minimal change in functional measures, treatment might shift to focus on skill-building or support in social reintegration. Using assessment results in this way ensures that treatment goals are both realistic and relevant, improving the likelihood of sustainable progress.

Using Baseline Data for Progress Monitoring

One of the key benefits of assessment tools is the ability to establish baseline measures that serve as reference points for tracking progress. Re-administering assessments at regular intervals enables clinicians to monitor changes, identify treatment effects, and adjust interventions accordingly. For example, if a patient's depression score decreases significantly but their quality of life score remains low, this might prompt a shift toward interventions focused on improving life satisfaction and social engagement.

Establishing progress markers based on assessment scores also provides clear, objective feedback for both the clinician and patient. Reviewing changes together helps patients see their improvement, which can enhance motivation and reinforce therapeutic engagement. This approach also supports clinicians in making evidence-based adjustments to the treatment plan, ensuring that care remains responsive to the patient's evolving needs.

Common Pitfalls in Assessment Interpretation and How to Avoid Them

Interpreting assessment results effectively requires awareness of potential pitfalls. Over-reliance on scores, for instance, can lead to a narrow view of the patient's condition, especially if assessments are not contextualized with qualitative information. It is also essential to recognize the limitations of each tool—no single assessment can capture all dimensions of a disorder. For example, a high score on an anxiety scale does not necessarily indicate an anxiety disorder; it could reflect anxiety related to an underlying mood or trauma disorder.

Another common pitfall is misinterpreting scores due to cultural or individual differences in symptom expression. A patient from a culture that discourages open expression of emotions may report lower symptom severity on self-report tools, even if they experience significant distress. Recognizing these nuances helps clinicians avoid underestimating symptoms and ensures that assessment interpretations remain culturally sensitive and individually tailored.

Integrating Results into the Diagnostic and Therapeutic Framework

Ultimately, assessment results should contribute to a comprehensive, multidimensional understanding of the patient. To do this, clinicians can:

- **Layer Quantitative Data with Qualitative Insights**: Combine scores with narrative data from interviews, observations, and self-reports to develop a full picture of the patient's experience.
- **Develop Hypotheses Based on Patterns**: Use assessment patterns to hypothesize about the primary drivers of the patient's difficulties and potential treatment barriers. For example, low motivation scores may signal a need for motivational interviewing techniques.

- **Collaborate with the Patient on Interpretation**: Involve the patient in understanding their results. Explaining what different scores mean, for example, in terms of symptom severity or functional impact, demystifies the diagnostic process and empowers patients to engage actively in treatment.

Integrating assessment results into the diagnostic and therapeutic framework enhances the clinician's ability to develop effective, individualized care plans. This approach not only ensures accurate diagnosis and appropriate treatment but also provides a structured, data-informed pathway for ongoing care and progress monitoring. Through careful interpretation of assessment results, clinicians can deliver a level of care that is not only responsive to current symptoms but also aligned with the patient's broader well-being and recovery goals.

Chapter 22: **Supplementary Online Resources**

Access our Virtual Assistant

Congratulations on reaching the end of this comprehensive guide to the DSM-5-TR and clinical diagnostics. We hope this resource has enriched your understanding and enhanced your diagnostic skills, providing practical strategies to apply in real-world settings.

With your purchase of this book, you gain exclusive access to a suite of supplementary online resources designed to support and extend your learning experience. Simply scan the QR code below to access the following benefits:

- **Expanded Interactive Questions**: Test your knowledge further with additional interactive questions across all major DSM-5-TR categories, developed to reinforce key concepts and support your diagnostic expertise.

- **Answer Guide for Interactive Chapters**: After logging in, receive complete answers and explanations for all interactive questions in the book, allowing for in-depth review and self-assessment.

- **Free Updates and New Exercises**: Stay current with ongoing updates, newly developed exercises, and diagnostic scenarios that reflect the latest research and clinical practices.

These supplementary tools are designed to keep your skills sharp, provide continuous learning, and support you in delivering high-quality, informed patient care.

Conclusion

As you complete this journey through the DSM-5-TR and the intricacies of clinical diagnosis, we hope you feel empowered and equipped to approach your work with confidence, insight, and empathy. This book is designed to be a comprehensive guide and a reliable companion as you navigate the complexities of mental health diagnostics, helping you make informed decisions that impact the lives of those you serve.

The landscape of mental health is ever-evolving, with new insights and understanding continuously shaping our approach to diagnosis and treatment. As you apply the principles and practices explored in this book, remember that your commitment to learning and growth is just as important as the tools and frameworks presented here. Each patient brings a unique story, and each case presents an opportunity to deepen your knowledge and refine your skills.

Whether you are a seasoned clinician or just beginning in this field, your role as a mental health professional holds immense value. The ability to diagnose with precision, offer meaningful guidance, and provide compassionate care transforms lives and builds healthier communities. We thank you for dedicating yourself to this work and hope this resource remains an invaluable tool on your path.

Remember to revisit these pages as often as you need, and take advantage of the supplementary resources available to you. Continue striving for excellence, seeking knowledge, and honoring the stories of each person who entrusts you with their care. Together, we contribute to a brighter future for mental health, one thoughtful diagnosis at a time.

Made in United States
Orlando, FL
16 February 2025

58415417R00125